Imported skin diseases

Imported skin diseases

editors

Prof.dr. W.R. Faber

Prof.dr. R.J. Hay

Dr. B. Naafs

ELSEVIER GEZONDHEIDSZORG, MAARSSEN

Online many more excellent images are available: see http://www.importedskindiseases.com.

This publication could not have been achieved without the support of the Q.M. Gastmann-Wichers Foundation.

Cover design: Mariël Lam, grafic design BNO, Empel.

Elsevier is an imprint of Reed Business Information bv, PO Box 1110, 3600 BC Maarssen,
The Netherlands.

To order: Elsevier Gezondheidszorg, Marketing dept., Antwoordnummer 2594 (freepost), 3600 VB
Maarssen, The Netherlands. Phone: +31-314-358358; fax: +31-346-577950;
e-mail: marketing.elseviergezondheidszorg@reedbusiness.nl or egz@reedbusiness.nl

ISBN-10   90 352 2804 9
ISBN-13   978 90 352 2804 9
NUR 876, 878

Editors and authors

Editors

Prof. William R. Faber MD PhD Dermatovenereologist
Study of Medicine University of Leiden, thereafter medical officer in Uganda, practiced as general practitioner in the Netherlands.Training for dermatovenereologist at the Binnengasthuis Amsterdam (prof.dr. R.H. Cormane), PhD University of Amsterdam. Thereafter consultant dermatologist at the Meander Medisch Centrum Amersfoort, and at the Academic Medical Center (AMC) Amsterdam.
At present Professor in Tropical Dermatology at the University of Amsterdam.

Prof. Roderick J. Hay DM FRCP FRCPATH
Head of the School of Medicine and Dentistry, Queen's University Belfast.
Professor Hay is an Honorary Consultant Dermatologist with the Belfast City Hospital Trust and Royal Hospitals Trust, Chairman of the International Foundation of Dermatology, Non Executive Director of the Eastern Health and Social Services Board. He holds an honorary Chair in the London School of Hygiene and Tropical Medicine.

Bernard Naafs MD PhD Dipl. TM&H Dermatovenereologist
Study of Medicine University of Utrecht, study of Tropical Medicine and Hygiene, Royal Tropical Institute (KIT) Amsterdam, thereafter Head clinical research All Africa Leprosy Rehabilitation and Training Centre (ALERT) Addis Ababa Ethiopia. Training for dermatovenereologist at the Binnengasthuis, Amsterdam (prof.dr. R.H. Cormane), PhD University of Amsterdam.
Head leprosy control Zimbabwe.
Head OPD Department of Dermatology Dijkzigt Hospital Erasmus University Rotterdam.
Thereafter consultant dermatologist IJsselmeerziekenhuizen Emmeloord/Lelystad. At present Consultant Tropical Dermatology at the Leiden University Medical Center (LUMC) in the Netherlands and visiting professor at the Regional Dermatology Training Centre (RDTC) Moshi Tanzania and at the Instituto Lauro de Souza Lima (ILSL) Bauru SP Brazil.

Authors per chapter

Acknowledgement
Secretarial support was given by Mrs. M. Schaap and technical and managerial support for the illustrations was supplied by Mr. R.R. Rodenburg.

Contents

1 Introduction

The world has developed into a global village in which people travel daily from continent to continent. Infectious diseases may travel the same way. Someone with an infection acquired under 'tropical' conditions abroad, may visit the health services in Europe or North-America within 24 hours of his or her departure from the country visited.

There are two main reasons why patients with 'tropical or exotic skin diseases' have been seen more frequently in recent years.

In the first place, in affluent societies leisure time is increasing, and more and more people, including those in the older age groups, take holidays in far-off places. More and more adventure holidays are taken to those places, where the risk of acquiring a disease is much greater than in a more protected environment.

In the second place, there are minority immigrant groups in most Western countries, originating from other continents. These people may regularly visit their family in their country of origin and acquire there a skin disease.

They may also present months or years after settling in their new home country.

Skin diseases are found in a considerable number of travellers. It is reported that among 2004 patients attending an Institute for Tropical Medicine in Berlin, Germany, 14% of the consultations were for skin diseases (1). From the United States of America a two year survey of 784 travellers to developing countries reported skin problems during travel in 8% of the travellers. In 3% of them these problems continued or had an onset within 14 days after return (2). Of 838 travellers to Nepal 12.44% were found to have skin diseases in which bacterial skin diseases, fungal skin diseases, scabies and 'skin allergy' were the most prevalent (3).

French researchers reported in a prospective study of French travellers to tropical countries, of whom 38% had visited Sub-Saharan Africa, that the most common diagnoses in 269 patients were cutaneous larva migrans (25%) and pyoderma (18%), followed by insect bites, myiasis, tungiasis, urticaria, fever and rash and cutaneous leishmaniasis in 10% or less. In 39% of the patients the skin lesions developed after the return to France. The median onset after departure from the tropics was 7 days (range 0-52 days) (4).

This book was written and illustrated for the health professional in order to help in the diagnosis and management of patients with diseases acquired in another, often tropical, environment. In this respect the book deals with skin diseases which do not usually exist in the Western world.

A wide spectrum of imported skin diseases, in the majority infectious in origin, is covered. Sexually transmitted infections as well as dermatological diseases are discussed.

Skin signs may provide the clue to the diagnosis of sometimes life-threatening-systemic infections; and should therefore be recognized as soon as possible by the attending physician. As travel these days is often not only terrestrial but also involves aqueous exposure in oceans or rivers a chapter on aquatic skin disorders is included.

The book also deals with emerging diseases such as cutaneous leishmaniasis, which is being diagnosed with increasing frequency in travellers and also in the military sector, and Buruli ulcer which is – still – rare in travellers.

The influence of environmental factors, the characteristics of pigmented skin, which influence the clinical expression of diseases in the coloured skin, and disorders of the pigmentary system itself are also addressed. Tables and flow charts of important clinical conditions and the relationship of those skin diseases to the different geographical areas will be helpful in the diagnosis and management of patients with imported skin diseases. Online many more excellent images are available: see http://www.importedskindiseases.com.

The contributions of the authors, all experts in their respective fields, are greatly appreciated.

REFERENCES
1   Harms G, Dorner F, Bienzle U, Stark K. Infections and diseases after travelling. *Dtsch Med Wochenschr* 2002;127:1748-53.
2   Hill DR. Health problems in a large cohort of Americans travelling to developing countries. *J Travel Med* 2000;7:259-66.
3   Caumes E, Brucker G, Brousse G, Durepaire R, Danis M, Gentilini M. Travel-associated illness in 838 French tourists in Nepal in 1984. *Travel Med Int* 1991;9:72-6.
4   Caumes E, Carriere J, Gwermonpieze G, Bricaire F, Danis M, Gentilini M. Dermatoses associated with travel to tropical countries: A prospective study of the diagnosis and management of 269 patients presenting to a tropical disease unit. *Clin Inf Dis* 1995;20:542-8.

2 Pigmentary disorders in black skin

J.P.W. van der Veen, M.F.E. Leenarts and W.W. Westerhof

2.1 INTRODUCTION

Western societies are becoming increasingly multiracial and all kinds of non-Caucasian skin types and mixed types can be seen nowadays, especially in the large metropolitan areas.

People with darker (non-white) skin types often seek medical attention for pigmentary problems that sometimes can be diagnosed as physiological for a particular skin type. On the other hand, in the dark skin, pathology often reflects in relative hyper- or hypopigmentation leading to specific clinical phenomena uncommon to white skin.

The colour of the skin is normally largely produced by the pigment melanin produced by the epidermal melanocytes and transferred to the epidermal keratinocytes.

In dark skin, melanocytes are larger and more dendritic, and produce larger melanosomes, which are being transferred in larger amounts to the epidermal keratinocytes.

At the same time, the pigment producing system is more vulnerable to noxious stimuli as can be observed in post-inflammatory hyper- and hypopigmentations.

Pigment problems can be very disturbing for patients with dark skin especially of course when huge contrasts with the constitutional skin colour emerge, such as can be seen in blacks with vitiligo.

Even objectively mild pigment problems however, can have important culturally determined psychosocial connotations in dark skinned patients and should therefore always be taken seriously by their doctors. In some areas pigment changes are easily associated with leprosy leading to social isolation of the persons involved.

In this chapter we will present you a concise overview of normal and abnormal pigmentations in dark skin.

2.2 NORMAL VARIATIONS IN ETHNIC SKIN

It is important to recognize normal pigmentary variations in dark skin in order to be able to reassure the patient and avoid unnecessary treatment.

A number of frequently seen conditions are described.

Voigt's or Futcher's lines

A total of five lines of demarcation between darker and lighter skin areas, the so-called Voigt's or Futcher's lines, have been described. These lines can be found on the upper arm anteromedially, the posterior portion of the lower limb, the presternal area, the posteromedial area of the spine, and the bilateral aspect of the chest. About 75% of the African-American population has at least one pigmentary demarcation line (1).

Hyperpigmentation at the extensor side of the joints (figure 2.1)

Stretching of the skin at the joints can possibly be a mechanical trigger for the melanocytes. Arthritis may also cause this hyperpigmentation (2).

Midline hypopigmentation

Midline hypopigmentation is characterized by hypopigmented, linear or discrete, ovoid macules occurring on the anterior aspect of the chest and the midsternal area. They can extend up to the chin and neck and down to the abdomen (3).

Figure 2.1 Hyperpigmentation at the extensor side of the joints

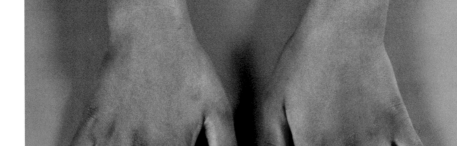

Nail pigmentation

Nail pigmentation manifests as longitudinal linear dark bands in the nail plate which occurs especially on the thumbs and index fingers (3). The pigmentation is usually absent at birth and increases with age. Nail pigmentation is mostly seen in blacks with a very dark complexion. It's important to differentiate these lesions from malignant melanoma and pigmentation secondary to drugs, chemicals and post-radiation changes (1).

Familial periorbital hyperpigmentation (figure 2.2)

Periorbital hyperpigmentation is a common finding in otherwise healthy people and has been described as an autosomal dominant hereditary disorder. The hyperpigmentation usually starts during childhood in the lower eyelids and progresses with age to involve the entire periorbital area (4). Periorbital hyperpigmentation can also be found in every skin type as an atopic stigma.

Linea nigra

The slightly pale linea alba, a line between the xyphoid process and the symphysis that in women normally can be observed on the abdomen, usually darkens during pregnancy and the more so in dark races leading to a so-called linea nigra.

Figure 2.2   Familial periorbital hyperpigmentation

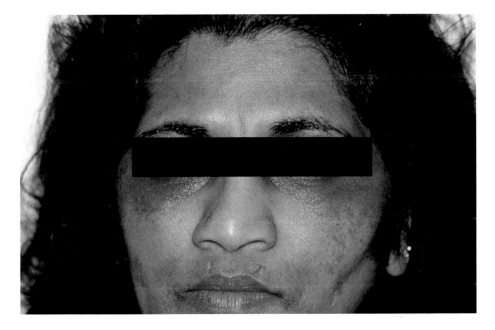

Oral pigmentation

Oral pigmentation is usually seen on the gingivae. The hard palate, buccal mucosa and tongue are less frequently involved. These lesions should be distinguished from conditions like secondary syphilis and drug eruptions. Unlike nail pigmentation, the skin colour cannot predict the likelihood of oral pigmentation (1).

Palmar and plantar hyperpigmentation

Macular hyperpigmentation is commonly seen on palms and soles of black patients. They vary in shape and are mottled in appearance. Clinically these must be differentiated from palmar/plantar lesions of syphilis, ephelides, nevi and melanoma.

Where in patients with fair skin pigmented lines in the palms can be a clinical future of M. Addison, this is a normal variation in people with dark skin (2).

Mongolian spot (figure 2.3)

This is the most common congenital hyperpigmentation, occurring in approximately 80 to 100% of the Asian and black newborns. It is a form of dermal melanocytosis in which melanocytes have been arrested in their fetal migration from the neural crest to the epidermis. The gray-blue macular lesions vary in size but usually occupy less than 5% of the body surface. The most common locations are the sacrum, buttocks and back.

Figure 2.3   Mongolian spot

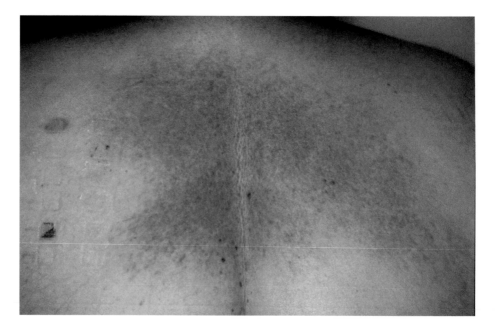

The majority of Mongolian spots intensify in colour during the first year of life followed by gradual disappearance. By the age of 10, virtually all Mongolian spots have disappeared (5).

2.3 ABNORMAL HYPER- AND HYPOPIGMENTATIONS

Nevus of Ota and nevus of Ito (figure 2.4)

These nevi are seen in all races, but affect mostly Asian people. Nevus of Ota or nevus fuscocoeruleus ophtalmomaxillaris is a dermal melanocytic hamartoma that presents as a bluish hyperpigmentation within the distribution of the first and second branch of the trigeminal nerve (6). Very often the sclerae are also involved. Histologically and clinically the lesions resemble Mongolian spots but are, unlike the latter condition, not self-limiting.

The pigmented spots usually appear in childhood and increase in number and extent to become confluent in some areas. The distribution is usually, but not always, unilateral. Malignant transformation has been reported in very rare instances. The nevus of Ito involves the acromioclavicular region and the upper chest and is similar to the nevus of Ota in its histology.

Both nevi have been reported to respond well to laser therapy, particularly the Q-switched ruby laser (7).

Figure 2.4   Nevus of Ota with eye involvement

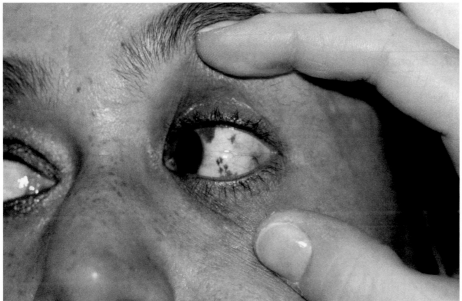

Transient neonatal pustular melanosis

Transient neonatal pustular melanosis (TNPM) can be seen in 2-5% of black new-borns.

The characteristic lesions consist of very superficial vesicopustules without any sign of erythema and ruptured pustules resulting in hyperpigmented papules with a surrounding collarette of scale in the first phase. Though always present at birth, the lesions can be easily overlooked and noticed for the first time several days after birth.

The lesions usually are 2 to 3 mm in diameter and can appear everywhere on the body, grouped or solitary. The head, neck, back, fingers and toes are predilection sites.

In the pustules neutrophils but no bacteria can be demonstrated.

The differential diagnosis of TNMP includes diseases like erythema toxicum and staphylococcal impetigo which can be differentiated by the typical clinical appearance and the history. The active vesiculopustules disappear in days, but the hyperpigmented macules slowly disappear in weeks to several months (5).

Ashy dermatosis

Ashy dermatosis or erythema dyschromicum perstans is seen worldwide but is most common in Latin America and Asia. It is seen somewhat more frequently in women than in men and has no age preference. Clinical manifestations include asymptomatic, slate-gray or violaceous hyperpigmented maculae distributed most commonly over the trunk and proximal extremities and less frequent over the face and neck. The maculae vary in size and shape and occasionally demonstrate an erythematous raised border in its early stages (8). The differential diagnosis should include lichen planus pigmentosus.

The etiology of ashy dermatosis remains unknown. At this time, no evidence-based treatment is available (9).

Dermatosis papulosa nigra (figure 2.5)

These small, darkly pigmented papules were originally described in African-Americans but are seen in darker-skinned people of many races. The incidence of this hereditary condition in black people rises from about 5% in the first decade to over 40% by the third, and is rather higher in females than in males.

The papules are often numerous in the malar regions and on the forehead and may occur on the neck and trunk. Treatment consists of diathermy or cautery (10).

Care has to be taken not to cauterize the normal surrounding skin in order to prevent the predictable induction of post-inflammatory hyperpigmentation.

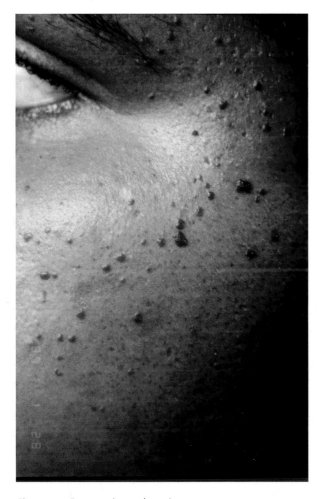

Figure 2.5   Dermatosis papulosa nigra

Pityriasis versicolor

Tinea versicolor or pityriasis versicolor is one of the most common pigmentary disorders worldwide. In tropical regions it is seen with a prevalence as high as 40%. It is s caused by overgrowth of commensal Malassezia yeasts, and affects most commonly the trunk. Patients have many slightly scaling macules and patches which can have, as implied by the name versicolor, many different colours such as yellowish-brown, pale yellow, or dark brown, occasionally reddish or pinkish, appearing hypopigmented or hyperpigmented (11). There is no correlation between pigmentary variation and skin colour (12).

Antifungal therapies usually cure the disease, but the pigment changes will disappear only slowly and recurrences can occur.

Melasma

Melasma is charactarized by irregular, usually symmetrical brown patches on sun-exposed skin. The malar prominences, the forehead, the upper lip, the nose and the chin are the most common sites of involvement but other areas like the neck and forearms can also be affected (13). Melasma is not exclusively a disorder of the darker skin types, but it appears to be far more common in Hispanics, Asians and Blacks. Etiologic factors include genetic and hormonal influences (pregnancy, birth control pills), exposure to UV-radiation, cosmetics, phototoxic drugs, and antiseizure medication. Current treatment options include the use of sunblocks, hypopigmenting agents and chemical peels.

Post-inflammatory hyperpigmentation

Post-inflammatory hyperpigmentation is one of the most common pigmentary disorders in dark skin. Inflammatory skin conditions like infections, bullous and pustular disorders, phototoxic eruptions, papulosquamous disorders, and medical interventions (laser therapy, chemical peels, dermabrasion) can all cause the increased pigmentation seen in post-inflammatory hyperpigmentation (13). The two processes involved are incontinentia pigmenti and an epidermal inflammatory response. Incontinentia pigmenti occurs after disruption of the epidermal basal cell layer causing dermal melanosis. The epidermal inflammatory response consists of an increased synthesis of melanin, resulting in an epidermal melanosis. The hyperpigmented areas correspond with the distribution of the original dermatosis. In this respect it is important to keep in mind that inflammatory disorders can present differently in dark skin as compared to white skin. Examples are the follicular atopic dermatitis and the papular pityriasis rosea. Blacks seem to have more follicular skin problems and post-acne hyperpigmentations in the face are very common. In epidermal melanosis the lesions are lighter brown and well-circumscribed, as compared to the darker gray, poorly circumscribed lesions in dermal melanosis. Dermal hyperpigmentation can take years to fade away to normal, whereas epidermal melanosis usually disappears in 6-12 months (14). Sun exposure, chemicals and certain drugs can aggravate post-inflammatory hyperpigmentation. The primary goal of therapy is treatment of the underlying inflammatory disease. Furthermore, treatment of post-inflammatory hyperpigmentation should always include the daily use of sunscreen. In addition, many topical agents have been used including keratolytics, retinoids, corticosteroids and depigmenting agents. Most significant improvement may be achieved by combining different agents.

Post-inflammatory hypopigmentation

Post-inflammatory hypopigmentation is caused by various cutaneous inflammatory diseases. The long use of potent corticosteroids, chemical peelings and medical interventions can also play a role. As in post-inflammatory hyperpigmentation, the configuration and distribution reflects the original dermatosis. In post-inflammatory hypopigmentation the melanocytes react with decreased melanin production after an inflammation or trauma. Sunlight exposure or photo (chemo) therapy may lead to repigmentation within months. Prevention of the trigger causing the hypopigmentation is important (15).

Pityriasis alba

Pityriasis alba is an eczematous disorder often occurring in children with an atopic background and dry skin. The lesions are typically hypopigmented, scaly, and asymptomatic and commonly affect the face but can also be seen on neck, arms and trunk. Most of the patients are children between 6 and 16 years of age. In many cases hardly noticeable on white skin, the disorder can be very conspicuous in black-skinned children. Sun exposure in conjunction with topical steroids and correction of the xerosis cutis is usually effective.

Idiopathic guttate hypomelanosis

One of the most common types of hypomelanosis in elderly people is idiopathic guttate hypomelanosis (IGH). An incidence of over 60% has been reported. IGH appears as numerous hypopigmented small macules (1-10 mm) on sun-exposed areas, such as the back of the hands, forearms, legs and occasionally on the face, abdomen and trunk (7). This dermatosis affects all races, is more frequent in women, and tends to increase in incidence with age. The etiology and pathogenesis are not well understood but since the lesions appear mainly on sun exposed areas, actinic damage may be a causal factor. No effective treatments are available (15).

Vitiligo

Vitiligo is characterized by the development of well-defined depigmented chalk white maculae, which can be present on any site of the body, but are usually seen on sites of stretch and pressure, in body folds and around body orifices (e.g. mouth).

Vitiligo occurs in all skin types and affects approximately 0.5% of the population world wide.

Understandingly, vitiligo in dark skinned patients is much more disfiguring than in whites. Due to the resemblance to leprosy, vitiligo patients in areas with endemic lepra often suffer from social exclusion.

The etiology remains unknown and several theories exist, such as the autoimmune hypothesis. The primary choice of treatment of vitiligo is UVB 311 nm light therapy. When vitiligo is stable, there are surgical treatment options, for example autologous minigrafting. If the depigmented lesions affect more than 80% of the body surface, complete depigmentation therapy can be considered (16).

Melanoma

Dark skin is better protected from sunlight, making sun-induced cancers less prevalent. Blacks have an incidence of malignant melanoma 5 to 18 times less than whites. However, at this moment there is a trend toward increased skin cancer rates in most ethnic groups (17). The prognosis of melanoma is related to the stage of the disease at the time of presentation. African-Americans diagnosed with melanoma have a worse prognosis than whites because they are initially seen with a more advanced disease.

Another significant difference is the primary tumor location. The most common melanoma location in African-Americans is the foot and in whites it is the trunk (18).

Progressive macular hypomelanosis

Progressive macular hypomelanosis is characterized by non-scaly, non-itchy, ill-defined hypopigmented macules on the skin. The macules occur on the front and the back of the trunk (less frequent on the face, the neck and the upper extremities) and are confluent in and around the midline. It occurs in young adults of both sexes but more often in women. Westerhof et al recently discovered follicular red fluorescence restricted to the hypopigmented spots. They proposed *Propionibacterium acnes* bacteria as a causing agent (19).

Final remarks

Regarding the vulnerability of dark skin to pigment changes, therapies intended to improve pigmentary problems should always be applied with great precaution.

All irritating agents or procedures have the potency of inducing post-inflammatory hyperpigmentation, so informing the patient and the use of small test areas are essential.

Primum non nocere should be our guideline.

REFERENCES

1   Mc Michael AJ. A review of cutaneous disease in African-American patients. *Dermatol Nursing* 1999;11(1):35-43.
2   Westerhof W, Menke HE. Pigmentproblemen in de donkere huid. In: Faber WR, Naafs B (eds.). Importdermatologie. Zeist: Glaxo BV, 1991;15-6.
3   Henderson AL. Skin variations in Blacks. *Cutis* 1983;32:376-7.
4   Ortonne JP, Bahadoran P, Fitzpatrick TB, Mosher DB, Hoi Y. Hypomelanoses and hypermelanoses. In: Fitzpatrick's Dermatology in General Medicine. 6th ed. Mc Graw-Hill; Vol 1, 2003;836-81.

5   Salmon JK, Frieden IJ. Congenital and genetic diseases of hyperpigmentation. In: Levine N (ed.). Pigmentation and pigmentary disorders, CRS Press, Boca Raton (FI) 1993;149-207.

6   Chan HH, Lam LK, Wong DS, Leung RS, Ying SY, Lai CF, et al. Nevus of Ota: a new classification based on the response to laser treatment. *Laser Surg Med* 20901;28:267-72.

7   Halder RM, Nandedkar MA, Neal KW. Pigmentary disorders in ethnic skin. *Dermatol Clin* 2003;21:617-28.

8   Schwartz RA. Erythema Dyschronicum perstans: the continuing enigma of Cinderella or Ashy dermatosis. *Int J Dermatol* 2004;43:230-2.

9   Kupres K, Meffert JJ. Ashy dermatosis. *Am Fam Physician* 2003;68(3):529-30.

10 Mac Kie RM, Quinn AG. Non-melanoma skin cancer and other epidermal skin tumours. In: Rook's textbook of dermatology. 7th ed. Blackwell Science Vol. 2. 2004;36-42.

11 Swartz RA. Superficial fungal infections. *Lancet* 2004;364:1173-82.

12 Aljabre SHM, Alzayir AAA, Abdulghani M, Osman OO. Pigmentary changes of tinea versicolor in dark-skinned patients. *Int J Dermatol* 2001;40:273-5.

13 Stratigos AJ, Katsambas AD. Optimal management of recalcitrant disorders of hyperpigmantation in dark-skinned patients. *Am J Clin Dermatol* 2004;5(3):161-8.

14 Lacz NL, Vafaie J, Kihicza NI, Schwartz RA. Postinflammatory hyperpigmentation: a common but troubling condition. *Int J Dermatol* 2004;43(5):362-5.

15 Hartmann A, Bröcker B, Becker JC. Hypopigmentary skin disorders. *Drugs* 2004;64(1):89-107.

16 Njoo MD. Treatment of vitiligo.Thesis, University of Amsterdam, 2000.

17 Halder MH, Ara CJ. Skin cancer and photoaging in ethnic skin. *Dermatol Clin* 2003;21:725-32.

18 Byrd KM, Wilson DC, Hoyler SS, Peck GL. Advanced presentation of melanoma in African Americans. *J Am Acad Dermatol* 2004;50: 21-4.

19 Westerhof W, Relyveld GN, Kingswijk MM, de Man P, Menke HE. Propionibacterium acnes and the pathogenesis of progressive macular hypomelanosis. *Arch Dermatol* 2004;40:210-4.

3 Coloured versus white skin

B. Naafs

3.1 INTRODUCTION

While in other medical specialities the clinical presentation of diseases hardly differs between the different races, in dermatology the aspect of a skin condition is certainly different in coloured skin than it is in white Caucasian skin. Skin diseases are expressed differently in different skins. For instance erythema, redness as a sign of inflammation – the hallmark of European-American dermatology – is difficult to appreciate in a pigmented skin. Pigment changes dominate the picture (1).

Races are different due to genetic differences, that manifest themselves in body build, form of head and face, length and shape of muscles and bones, but even more in the colour of the skin, and the colour and form of the hair. Until recently most publications on ethnic differences in dermatology were not well researched and did not make allowances for different climatic or socio-economic circumstances (2,3,4). But more and more it has become clear that some of the differences are important because they influence the clinical presentation of skin diseases.

The major differences between coloured skin and white skin are in (1,2,3,4,5):
- the clinical expression of erythema.
- the de-, hypo- and hyperpigmentation of darker skins.
- the larger cohesion between the keratinocytes in the coloured skin.
- a greater tendency of the coloured skin to lichenification.
- a greater tendency to keloid formation in the non-white skin.
- a greater risk of epidermal skin cancers in the white skin.

3.2 ERYTHEMA

Due to the overlying pigmentation, erythema, a sign of inflammation, is not easily visible in a black skin (figure 3.1). Therefore palpation is even more important in the examination of pigmented skin than it is in white skin. During palpation the other signs of inflammation, calor (heat, warmth), tumor (swelling) and dolor (pain, tenderness) can be appreciated. Sometimes erythema may manifest as a dark violet hue. The condition erythroderma is not clearly visible as such in the black skin and can only be seen as an exfoliative dermatitis.

B

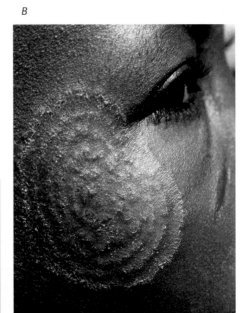

A

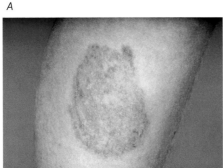

Figure 3.1   A, B Tinea imbricata, absence of erythema in black skin

3.3 PIGMENT CHANGES

Pigment changes (de-, hypo- and hyperpigmentation) dominate the clinical picture in the dermatology of the pigmented skin (1,6).

Depigmentation can be seen during the extreme desquamation that may occur when psoriasis is treated aggressively, or when there is a total disruption in the transfer of melanosomes, as happens in some forms of cutaneous lupus erythematosus (figure 3.2). The melanocyte itself can disappear due to cytotoxicity in autoimmune diseases such as vitiligo or as a result of toxic substances as seen in some leucodermas (cheap rubber).

Hypopigmentation can be due to an increased desquamation of the skin. The turnover of keratinocytes is increased, whereas the pigment synthesis is not, so that each keratinocyte contains less pigment. In an epidermis of the same thickness this results in hypopigmentation. This can be seen in pityriasis alba, which is probably a mild form of atopic dermatitis, and in post-inflammatory hypopigmentation. Another phenomenon that may occur is that the transfer of melanosomes from the melanocyte to the keratinocytes is hindered by edema and inflammatory cells, as may occur in eczema (spongiotic dermatitis), or by down regulation of PAR-2, a protease-activated receptor (PAR) involved in melanosome uptake from the melanocyte

A 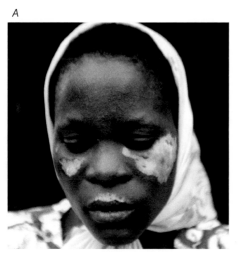 B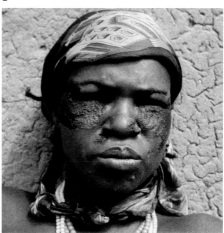

Figure 3.2 A, B Discoid lupus erythematosus: in one patient depigmentation in the other hyperpigmentation

into the keratinocyte (6). A third possibility is that the pigment synthesis itself is suppressed. This seems the case in the hypopigmented variant of pityriasis versicolor where the yeast Malassezia suppresses melanin synthesis and in tuberculoid leprosy, where the synthesis may be inhibited by autoimmunity. Also toxic substances like phenolic detergents may diminish pigmentation.

Topical steroids cause hypopigmentation by two mechanisms: the steroid suppresses pigment formation and the epidermis becomes thinner.

Hyperpigmentation can be seen when the epidermis is thickened as in lichenification or in untreated psoriasis which present with a thicker layer of keratinocytes, each keratinocyte with its share of pigment. Sometimes infectious agents cause hyperpigmentation; in the dark variant of pityriasis versicolor, large melanosomes can be seen. Pigment incontinence is a third important cause. In many of the inflammatory conditions the basement membrane loses its integrity and pigment leaks into the dermis where it is phagocytized by phagocytes e.g. melanophages. Such pigment appears to be blue-black (a pigmented particle always seems blue when it is located deep in the dermis) and disappears only very slowly, e.g. post-inflammatory hyperpigmentation.

One should be aware that while the same dermatosis might lead to hyperpigmentation in one patient, in an other it may cause hypo- or even depigmentation (figure 3.2). Even in a single person the same disease may lead to difference in pigmentation.

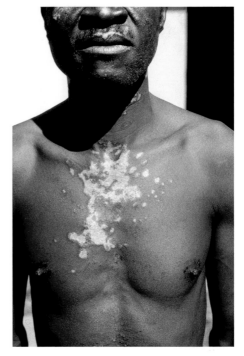

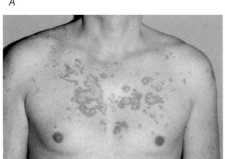

Figure 3.3 A, B Subacute cutaneous lupus erythematosus: distribution, localisation and configuration are the same

Although dermatoses appear different in different races, their distribution, localisation and configuration are the same, which may be helpful in establishing the clinical diagnosis (figure 3.3) (1).

3.4 COHESION

The cohesion between keratinocytes in pigmented skin is stronger than in white skin (1,4). Therefore, while scratching a Caucasian skin leads to excoriation and exudative skin lesions, in the pigmented skin lichenification often occurs, especially in the mongoloid skin where it may show as a grey hue. In the black skin, where lichenification is also common, there is often a tendency to develop follicular lesions. This follicular lichenification is often misdiagnosed as lichen nitidus even by an experienced dermatologist.

In comparison with white skin, the stratum corneum in black skin is equal in thickness but more compact, about 16 layers are seen in white versus 20 layers in black skin, probably due to the greater cohesion between the keratinocytes.

A

B

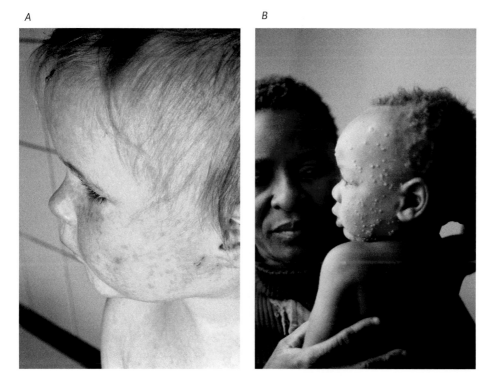

Figure 3.4   A, B Varicella: in white skin vesicles are broken, in black skin intact

Therefore, while in white skin vesicles break easily, in black skin they remain intact (figure 3.4). As a result herpes and varicella lesions remain for a long time in dark skin; and 'eczematous dermatitis' in this pigmented skin is not wet and polymorphic, but papular and lichenified. These papules in fact are vesicles, because a vesicle in black skin is frequently not appreciated as a vesicle but, due to the overlying pigment, may be considered to be a papule. Papular eczema is typical for the coloured, especially the black, skin and is often not recognised as such. One should realise that, though the macroscopic aspects differ, histopathologically the diseases are the same – spongiotic dermatitis.

Blisters especially in intra-epidermal bullous diseases (e.g. pemphigus) in dark skin are larger than the blisters in the white Caucasian skin, again due to the larger cohesion between the keratinocytes in the coloured skin, especially in the stratum corneum. However, Nikolsky's sign, which is related to a near absent cohesion within the epidermis, remains a useful test also in black skin.

3.5 KELOID FORMATION

Coloured skin tends to keloid formation. Even minimal stimuli may induce this (figure 3.5). It especially happens in the neck, on the earlobes, on the shoulders, back, and presternal area, the area normally covered by a stola. But it may occur anywhere. A good explanation for keloid formation is not yet available.

3.6 PIGMENTATION AND SKIN CANCER

Since the number of melanocytes are equal in all skin types, it is the nature, quantity and distribution of the melanosomes, the organelles that contain the melanin, in the epidermis that play a crucial role in the determination of skin colour and the skin's

Figure 3.5   Keloids

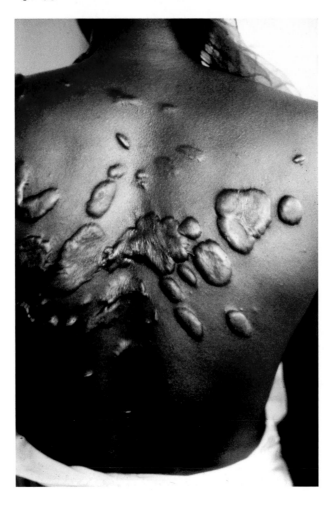

sensitivity to UV radiation. In Caucasian skin the melanosomes are small and oval and aggregated in groups of three or more within a membrane situated like an umbrella above the nucleus of the keratinocyte. When keratinocytes move up towards the stratum corneum, the melanosomes are broken up. In Negroid skin they are larger and more rounded and are lying dispersed within keratinocytes and stay intact up to the stratum corneum. They contain two types of melanin, black and brown eumelanin, and reddish-brown pheomelanin. Eumelanin gives a better protection against UV light than pheomelanin.

Pigmentation protects against skin cancers that result from UV damage to the DNA (2). It has been shown in vitro that in light skinned individuals the in presence of L-tyrosine increased melanin production leads to a more elliptical shape of the melanosomes. X-ray microanalyses of these melanosomes showed that in melanocyte cultures of light skinned individuals there was a larger increase in sulphur content of the melanosomes than in that of the dark skinned. HPLC analysis showed the ratio between pheomelanin and eumelanin was found to increase more markedly in light skin derived melanocytes than in those from the dark skin (7). Pheomelanin production is a thiol-consuming process and may lead to an increased risk of oxidative stress in these cells and hence an increased cancer risk. This observation together with the limited ability of pheomelanin to absorb UV radiation may also contribute to the higher skin cancer risk in the light skinned individual especially among the Celtic phenotype, which has a predominance of pheomelanin.

3.7 OTHER DIFFERENCES

Most physical properties are not well researched. There are studies that suggest that the transepidermal water loss (TEWL) is greater in Negroid than in Caucasian skin and there is an observation that desquamation of Negroid skin is greater than that of Caucasian and Mongoloid skin (3). This may account for the xerosis so often encountered in Negroid skin.

It is observed that black skin is more resistant to irritants. This probably can be explained by the fact that the stratum corneum of black individuals is more compact and consists, though of same thickness, out of more layers.

Microscopic evaluation reveals that Negroid skin contains larger mast cell granules than Caucasian skin (3). It is tempting to speculate that this accounts for the observation that black patients report pruritis more frequently than other ethnic groups. Though xerosis may also be an important cause.

A pure physical property of the colour of the black skin is that, especially in radiated heat, (the sun), it absorbs more heat than a lighter coloured or white skin, resulting in more sweating in the dark coloured individual. Contrary to what is often said, the density of eccrine sweat glands of black and white is the same. There may be some differences in the apocrine glands between the different ethnic groups, less dense in East Asians more in Africans (4). In the cold black skin radiates more heat, hence the tendency of black people to dress in warm clothes and to cover themselves at night. In particular they cover their head where the closely-cropped hair allows the warmth to escape easily.

3.8 HAIR

Hair differs in distribution, colour and form among different ethnic groups (1,4). Caucasians of Mediterranean origin or Turkish or Iranian extraction may be extensively hairy, in contrast to Nordic Caucasians, Indians and Mongoloids. The hair colour of Negroids, Mongoloids and Australoids is almost always black, while the colour of Caucasian hair varies from deep black to blonde or reddish. The hair of Mon-

Figure 3.6   Traction alopecia

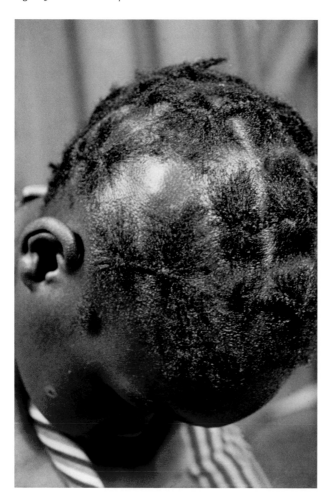

goloids and Negroids is thick, that of Caucasians usually thin. The hair of Negroids is stiff and curly, that of Mongoloids straight, while that of Caucasians is straight or wavy. Negroid hair is oval, that of the other races more rounded. The hairs leave the skin at an angle of 90 degrees in white individuals but with a sharp angle in black individuals.

Curly stiff hairs may cause problems, especially after shaving when the hairs curl inside the skin and cause inflammation, as is seen in pseudofolliculitis barbae and acne cheloidalis nuchae.

The distribution of Negroid and Mongoloid hair is often less dense than that in Caucasians. There is some indication that the anchoring of Negroid hair is less strong, which may explain in part traction alopecia that is so often encountered in black patients. Also their hair seems to be more brittle. But these observations must be weighed against the cosmetic manipulations where curly hair in black people is often subjected to, e.g. straightening, weaving and knotting (figure 3.6).

REFERENCES

1   Naafs B. De blanke en de gekleurde huid. *Ned Tijdschr Dermatol Venereol* 1999;9:247-53.
2   Taylor SC. Skin of color: biology, structure, function, and implications for dermatologic disease. *J Am Acad Dermatol* 2002;46(2 Suppl.):S41-62.
3   Wesley NO, Maibach HI. Racial (ethnic) differences in skin properties: the objective data. *Am J Clin Dermatol* 2003;4:843-60.
4   Gawkrodger DJ. Racial influences on skin disease. In: Burns T, Breathnach S, Cox N, Griffiths C (eds.). Rook's textbook of dermatology, London (UK): Blackwell Publishing 2004:69.1-69.21.
5   Berardesca E, Maibach H. Ethnic skin: overview of structure and function. *J Am Acad Dermatol* 2003;48 (6 Suppl.):S139-42.
6   Seiberg M. Keratinocyte-melanocyte interactions during melanosome transfer. *Pigment Cell Res* 2001;14(4):236-42. Review.
7   Nieuwpoort F van, Smit NP, Kolb R, Van der Meulen H, Koerten H, Pavel S. Tyrosine-induced melanogenesis shows differences in morphologic and melanogenic preferences of melanosomes from light and dark skin types. *J Invest Dermatol* 2004;122(5):1251-5.

4 Influence of old and new environment on the skin

Environmental related skin disorders in immigrants and tourists

H.E. Menke

4.1 INTRODUCTION

This chapter is about skin disorders which are induced by the change in environment. We shall discuss skin diseases in immigrants from (sub)tropical countries to the temperate climatic zone and in tourists returning home from the (sub)tropics to the temperate climatic zone. We shall focus especially on disorders which are probably related to the new environment or to be more precise: to lack of adaptation to the new environment. For the immigrant the temperate climatic zone and for the tourist the (sub)tropical climatic zone is the new environment. This is in fact a broad subject with unfortunately a relative paucity of medical publications. In this chapter we shall discuss only a few disorders as an example of this topic. For detailed information we refer the reader to textbooks and special articles.

In immigrants from (sub)tropical countries moving to the temperate climatic zone as well as in tourists returning home to the temperate climatic zone, after a vacation in a (sub)tropical country, a myriad of infectious as well as non-infectious skin disorders can be encountered. Most of these conditions are however non-infectious by nature. Some are related to the racial background or ethnicity of the individual. Skin disorders peculiar to certain ethnic groups are nowadays designated as ethnic skin disorders. Ethnicity is a concept different from race. It is used for several reasons, including the fact that some groups of people do not fit easily into a race. It is actually an imprecise concept, which implies shared origins including cultural traditions that are maintained between generations, leading to a sense of identity in a group (1). Many ethnic skin disorders are diseases of pigmentation and discussed in chapter 2. Non-pigmentary ethnic skin disorders are numerous, examples of which are lichen amyloidosis, common in Chinese people and keloid, seen especially in people from African descent. Most ethnic skin disorders are common in the countries of origin, so they are not specifically related to migration.

4.2 ENVIRONMENT, ADAPTATION AND SKIN DISORDERS

Skin disorders can be induced by environmental factors, which can be subdivided in:

1   Physical factors, e.g. sunlight including UV radiation, ambient temperature (heat, cold), and degree of humidity (moistness, dryness).
2   Biological factors, e.g. micro organisms, animals and plants.
3   Factors produced by the industrialized societies, which are absent or uncommon in a non-industrialized environment, e.g. toxic chemical agents (2).

Other factors determining the development of skin diseases are structure and function of the skin, immunological factors and finally social, cultural and psychological factors, including behaviour. An example of a skin disease related to the latter group of factors is exogenous ochronosis, an unwanted side effect of the (mis)use of bleaching creams containing hydroquinone.

Structure and function of the skin in people originating from tropical countries, are in some respects different from those of people from a temperate, less sunny climate (3). Molecular analysis has identified genetic differences between races and ethnic groups, probably related to differences in their environment. Most anthropologists believe that racial variation developed through natural selection processes: different biologic traits in the races developed because these traits facilitated adaptation to a particular environment. For instance, it is believed that darkly pigmented skin evolved to protect those people living close to the equator from ultraviolet (UV) light. People living north of the equator on the other hand, probably have paler skin to ensure adequate absorption of UV rays to promote vitamin D formation in the basal layer of the epidermis. Besides the difference in skin colour, there are other anatomical differences in the skin between people from diverse regions of the earth. For example, dark skinned people probably have larger apocrine sweat glands and in greater numbers than white subjects. The stratum corneum of black people is more compact than that of white people, reflecting a stronger intercellular cohesion, and this could be responsible for the fact that continuous scratching in black people often leads to lichenification. However, racial differences have been minimally investigated by objective methods and the data are often contradictory (4).

The immune system, including the so-called skin immune system, plays a major role in defending the body against microbial intruders. In a new environment with micro-organisms in the ecosystem which are immunologically unknown to the traveller or immigrant, infectious diseases including skin infections can develop, which would not appear in the old environment. According to the so-called hygiene theory, epidemiological and laboratory studies have implied that the environment during early childhood is important for the risk of developing atopic disorders. The prevalence of asthma, hay fever and eczema among 1901 internationally adopted boys in Sweden was analyzed in relation to indicators of their early childhood environment. The adopted males who came to Sweden before two years of age suffered from asthma, hay fever and eczema significantly more often than those who came to Sweden between 2 and 6 years of age. This study demonstrates that environment during the first years of life has a profound influence on the risk of suffering from atopic disorders as young adults (5).

In conclusion, from the above mentioned examples it should be clear that the interaction between factors present in a certain climatic zone on the one hand and biological traits and behaviour of the individual on the other hand, can induce 'new' skin disorders in individuals coming from another climatic zone.

4.3 SKIN DISORDERS IN IMMIGRANTS

In this paragraph we shall describe some examples of skin disorders in immigrants from (sub)tropical countries to the temperate climatic zone, due to the change of environment.

4.3.1 Dry skin and dry eczema

Dry skin or xerosis is one of the most common skin disorders in people coming from a warm humid tropical climate to a temperate climate. It is one of the skin disorders related to the humidity level (table 4.1). Dry skin and eczema can develop very soon after arrival, especially during wintertime. These disorders are more common in people taking frequent hot and long showers and using soap excessively.

The natural 'oily coating' on top of and within the horny layer of the epidermis, called 'natural skin emulsion' is composed of an oily component and a watery component, produced by the skin itself. If this coating disappears, the skin loses water and may

Table 4.1 Skin diseases related to the degree of humidity

Dry environment

itch

dry skin

ichthyosiform skin

cracquelé type eczema

Humid (and hot) environment

miliaria

bacterial infections (pyoderma)

fungal and yeast infections

develop signs of the dry skin syndrome. These range from mild to severe and are successively: a dry scaly skin, an ichthyosiform skin and a cracquelé eczema, characterized by nummular patches of slight erythema, a mild infiltration, cracks and scaling (figure 4.1). If the skin is dark, the erythema cannot be identified. The accompanying symptoms are a 'dry feeling', itching (sometimes severe and even disturbing sleep) and sometimes pain. The disorder can be localized anywhere on the body, but most common are legs and arms, but also the face, especially the lips can be affected.

The diagnosis is easy to make on clinical grounds. It must however be differentiated from other types of eczema, e.g. contact dermatitis and atopic dermatitis. Signs and symptoms of other skin conditions can be worsened by dry skin. Complications of dry skin can be infection and lichenification.

The disorder can be treated with a class 1 or 2 corticosteroid (hydrocortisone or triamcinolone) containing fatty ointment, to be used for a short time, only if eczema is present. An emollient or an urea containing cream can be used as maintenance therapy.

Finally it is important to give the patient bathing and general advices: decrease the frequency and duration of showering; use warm, not hot water; do not use soap; dry the skin gently with a towel, patting is better than rubbing; use a hydrating ointment after drying the skin. Finally, it can be worthwhile to use a humidifier in the home if the air is very dry.

Figure 4.1   Dry cracquelé eczema

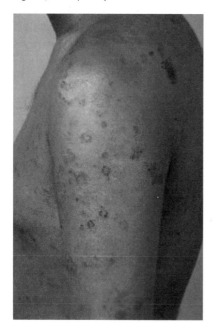

Figure 4.2   Chickenpox

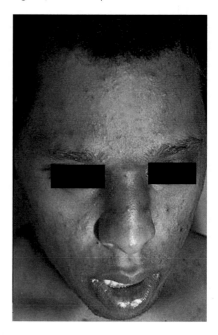

4.3.2 Chickenpox (varicella)

Chickenpox or varicella is a very contagious disease, caused by the varicella/zoster virus. The disease is spread by droplet airborne transmission. The incubation time is between 10 and 21 days. After a prodromal phase of 2 or 3 days with fever, malaise and flu like symptoms, the skin eruption appears (figure 4.2). Lesions often begin on the face/head region and than spread. Lesions in the mouth and vagina are common. The initial lesion on a white skin is an erythematous macule, followed by a small vesicle, which later transforms in a pustule, subsequently an erosion and finally a scab. The lesions appear in crops, with new crops appearing for an average of 3-4 days. Total healing takes 2 to 3 weeks. The eruption can be extremely itchy. On a dark skin the initial erythematous macules are obscure and after healing 'polka dot' hyper-pigmented scars can be present for many months and sometimes even years.

The disease is usually mild, but serious complications can occur. These include secondary bacterial infection of the skin, otitis media, pneumonitis and encephalitis.

The differential diagnosis with insect bites can cause problems. Typical prodromal symptoms and lesions on mucosal membranes can be helpful in making the right diagnosis.

A definite diagnosis can be made by isolating the virus from a lesion or by antibody assessment.

Antiviral drugs like aciclovir and valaciclovir are effective and should be considered for adolescents and individuals with eczema.

Chickenpox is very common in certain immigrant groups coming from (sub)tropical countries to Europe or the United States. In a group of Tamil refugees to Denmark, 38% of the adults and 68% of the children developed chickenpox in the first few months after arrival, due to lack of immunity (6). Struewing et al (7) suggest that members of a high-risk immigrant group could benefit from varicella vaccination.

4.3.3 Perniosis (chilblains)

This is typical a disorder of wintertime, caused by an abnormal vascular reaction to cold in probably genetically predisposed persons. It is a common disorder. Other examples of cold induced skin disorders are listed in the table 4.2.

Immigrants from (sub)tropical countries, not using gloves and wearing inadequate footwear in the cold season are prone to perniosis. The clinical signs are red or purple patches on the feet and/or hands, sometimes with infiltration and even blisters and necrosis (figure 4.3). The symptoms are pain and itch. It must be differentiated from other diseases with similar symptoms, like chilblain lupus erythematosus, a variant of systemic lupus erythematosus and lupus pernio, a variant of sarcoidosis.

Table 4.2 Skin diseases caused (or deteriorated) by cold

perniones (chilblains)

livedo reticularis

Raynaud's phenomenon

cold panniculitis

cryoglobulinaemia

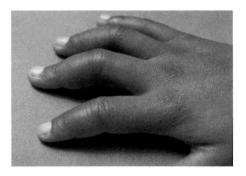

Figure 4.3 Perniones

The treatment is difficult. One should advice adequate gloves, footwear and ambient temperature. Vasodilating drugs might be of some use (8).

4.3.4 Psoriasis

Lack of exposure to sunlight (visible and/or ultraviolet) in immigrants in Europe, coming from sunny (sub)tropical countries can induce or provoke diseases that would not have appeared if they had remained in their old environment. Examples (based on epidemiological studies and case reports) are seasonal mental depression (9) and osteomalacia and rickets (10). Based on his own experience as a dermatologist in the Netherlands, the author has the impression that psoriasis might be another example. However, further investigation is needed to substantiate this idea.

Psoriasis is a common genetically determined chronic relapsing skin disorder, clinically characterised by (in the white skin) the presence of sharply delineated patches with erythema, thickening and scaling.

Its worldwide prevalence is between approximately 1-3%, although it appears to be uncommon in certain populations like for example South American Indians. It is suggested that it is less common in people from African descent than in Europeans.

In people with ethnic skin, the disease has the same clinical characteristics as in whites, although the erythema is obscured by pigmentation (figure 4.4).

After healing, a typical hypopigmented spot remains which slowly repigments. The typical localisations of lesions are the extensor sides of knees and elbows, the sacral region and the scalp, but lesions can appear on virtually any part of the body. The lesions are not or slightly itchy. The clinical characteristics are usually sufficient to enable the diagnosis to be made. Lesions in dark skinned people can sometimes cause difficulties in making the right diagnosis. Eczema, especially nummular eczema , can resemble psoriasis; the same is true for neurodermatitis circumscripta (lichen simplex), lichen planus and parapsoriasis. A skin biopsy for histological

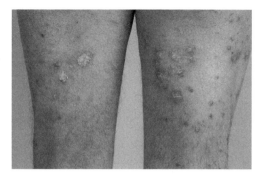

Figure 4.4   Psoriasis

investigation can sometimes be helpful in making the right diagnosis. People coming from (sub)tropical countries can have their first episode of psoriasis after coming to Europe. One can speculate that the lack of UV light (which normally suppresses the disease) in the new environment, might be responsible. Psychological stress related with the life in the new environment, is another hypothetical explanation.

The treatment for psoriasis is diverse and we refer to textbooks of dermatology.

4.4 SKIN DISORDERS IN TOURISTS
In this paragraph we shall discuss some examples of skin disorders in tourist coming home to the temperate climatic zone after a holiday in the (sub)tropics.

4.4.1 Miliaria
Miliaria or prickly heat is a disorder caused by blocking of the ducts of the eccrine sweat glands, probably caused by common skin bacteria like *Staphylococcus epidermidis* and *Staphylococcus aureus*. It is possible that the obstruction develops easy in people from a temperate climate zone in whom the function of sweating is less developed. Three types of miliaria are recognized, related to the level of the obstruction:

1   Miliaria crystallina: in this case the obstruction is in the stratum corneum, causing tiny superficial blisters with clear fluid, that easily rupture. The disorder is asymptomatic.
2   Miliaria rubra: this is the most common type; here the blocking is in the epidermis, causing itchy or stinging erythematous or skin coloured non follicular papules and papulovesicles (figure 4.5).
3   Miliaria profunda: the blocking is at the level of the dermo-epidermal junction causing itchy skin coloured non follicular papules.

Miliaria is a common disorder in tourists visiting a hot humid climate, developing within a few days after arrival. The lesions are localized especially on the trunk, but

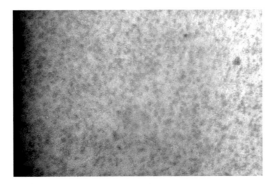

Figure 4.5   Miliaria rubra

can also be found on the head and neck region and the extremities. Complications are secondary bacterial infection, causing miliaria pustulosa or other types of pyoderma and disturbed heat regulation. Sweating is the most important means of heat regulation in a hot environment and blocking of sweating can cause body temperature to rise, causing a heat stroke with thirst, dizziness, weakness and high body temperature.

Miliaria is generally easily diagnosed. It must be differentiated from folliculitis, which is characterized by follicular localized papules and pustules.

A cool bath or cool (air-conditioned) environment are excellent general measures. Miliaria crystallina is a self-limiting disorder not requiring special other measures. Miliaria rubra and profunda can be treated topical with antipruritic agents. The disorder normally disappears within some days after arrival in a cooler climate.

4.4.2 Sunburn (dermatitis solaris)

Sunburn is an acute inflammatory reaction of the skin, caused by the direct effect of light, which can start as soon as 30 minutes after sun exposition, characterized by erythema, swelling (edema), vesicles, bullae and erosions of the sun exposed region. The symptoms are a burning feeling, tenderness and pain which can be extreme. If a large area of the body is involved, it can be accompanied by systemic symptoms like fever, malaise, nausea and vomiting, dizziness, lowering of blood pressure and shock. It can be complicated by secondary bacterial infection. Sunburn is caused by ultraviolet radiation, especially UVB (290-320 nm). It is more common close to the equator and at high altitudes. Lighter skinned individuals (skin phototype I-III) are more frequently and severely affected than darker skinned types.

Diagnosis is easy on clinical grounds. The treatment consists of cool compresses, and anti-inflammatory medication like topical or systemic corticosteroids or NSAIDs.

Table 4.3   Skin diseases caused by sunlight including UV radiation

sunburn (dermatitis solaris)
polymorphic light eruption
solar urticaria
actinic prurigo
phototoxic reactions
photoallergic reactions

Sunburn can be prevented by avoiding sun exposure, wearing of protective clothing and the regular use of sunscreens with an adequate SPF (30 or higher).

Sunburn is by far the most common light induced disorder occurring during a holiday in the (sub)tropics, but a number of other photodermatoses may develop (see table 4.3).

Finally some pre existing skin disorders can exacerbate or aggravate during sun exposure, for example herpes simplex and lupus erythematosus.

REFERENCES

1   Marmot MG. General approaches to migrant studies: the relation between disease, social class and ethnic origin. In: Cruickshank JK, Beevers DG (eds.). Ethnic Factors in Health and Disease. London: Wright, 1989;12-7.

2   English JSC, Dawe RS and Ferguson, J. Environmental effects and skin diseases. *British medical Bulletin* 2003;68:129-42.

3   Taylor SC. Skin of color: Biology, structure, function, and implications for dermatologic disease. *J Am Acad Derm* suppl. 2002;46:S41-62.

4   Wesley ON and Maibach HI. Racial (ethnic) differences in skin properties. The objective data. *Am J Clin Dermatol* 2003;4 (12):843-60.

5   Hjern A, Rasmussen F, Hedlin G. Age at adoption, ethnicity and atopic disorder: a study of internationally adopted young men in Sweden. *Pediatr Allergy Immunol* 1999;10:101-6.

6   Kjersem H, Jepsen S. Varicella among immigrants from the tropics, a health problem. *Scand J Soc Med* 1990;18:171-4.

7   Struewing JP, Hyams KC, Tueller JE, Gray GC. The risk of measles, mumps, and varicella among young adults; a serosurvey of US Navy and Marine Corps recruits. *Am J Public Health* 1993;83:1717-20.

8   Rustin MHA, Newton JA, Smith MP et al. The treatment of chillblains with nifedipine. *Br J Dermatol* 1989;120:267-75.

9   Suhail K, Cochrane R. Seasonal changes in affective state in samples of Asian and white women. *Soc Psychiatr Epidemiol* 1997;32:149-57.

10 Wauters IMPMJ en van Soesbergen RM. Ziek door te weinig zonlicht: rachitis en osteomalacie. *Ned Tijdschr Geneeskd* 1999;143:593-7.

5 Fungal infections

R.J. Hay

5.1 INTRODUCTION

Fungal infections or mycoses that affect the skin include some of the commoner of human diseases ranging from tinea pedis or athlete's foot to cutaneous manifestations of deep infections, sometimes rare and, occasionally, life threatening (1). The latter include diseases such as cryptococcosis that occur in HIV positive patients, during which blood stream dissemination to the skin may occur. Imported infections may be seen in all of these categories, although clinical presentation may occur years after the individual has left his country of origin. As with all potentially imported disease there are patients who present with infections after a short visit to a tropical environment, because an existing infection has been exacerbated by the different climatic conditions; equally there are those who acquire a new infection as a result of their residence overseas.

There are three main groups of fungal infection, the superficial, subcutaneous and systemic infections (table 5.1).

The superficial infections are world wide in distribution, although there are regional variations, and they include the dermatophyte or ringworm infections, superficial candidosis or thrush and *Malassezia* infections of which the common skin disease, pityriasis versicolor, is an example. The subcutaneous mycoses, with some exceptions, are largely confined to the tropics and subtropics; here the infection is usually introduced by implantation of the organisms from the external environment. These infections are largely confined to the subcutaneous tissue and dermis but may extend to the epidermis as well as bone. They may present with skin manifestations. The systemic infections involve deep structures. Some are primarily respiratory and infection follows inhalation. The skin is affected if there is blood stream spread or, more rarely, if the infection is directly introduced into the skin. In the opportunistic systemic fungal infections the organisms gain entry via different routes e.g. gastrointestinal tract, intravenous catheters, but blood stream spread to the skin is possible. In these many of these systemic mycoses involvement of the skin is variable and unpredictable. However some infections affecting patients with AIDS are highly

Table 5.1   Classification of mycoses and the main imported infections

Superficial mycoses	
dermatophytosis	tinea capitis; rare: tinea imbricate
superficial candidosis	
disease due to *Malassezia*	
others e.g. *Scopulariopsis* infections	infection due to *Scytalidium*
Subcutaneous mycoses	
mycetoma	all are uncommon imported diseases – in Europe mycetoma and phaeohyphomycosis are probably the two most frequently encountered of the subcutaneous mycoses
chromoblastomycosis	
phaeohyphomycosis	
others e.g. infection due to *Conidiobolus* or *asidiobolus*	
Systemic mycoses	
Endemic mycoses	
histoplasmosis	all endemic systemic mycoses can be seen as imported diseases – in Europe the most frequent is histoplasmosis
blastomycosis	
coccidioidomycosis	
paracoccidiodomycosis	
infection due to *Penicillium marneffei*	these can occur in any environment
Opportunistic mycoses	
systemic candidosis	
aspergillosis	
zygomycosis	
cryptococcosis	
others e.g. *Fusarium, Trichosporon*	

likely to show cutaneous involvement, e.g. infections due to *Penicillium marneffei* and these may also present in travellers who have visited an endemic area for a comparatively short time.

The pathogenic fungi usually exist as chains of cells, hyphae, or single cells that reproduce by budding, yeasts, in human tissue. Fungi are said to be dimorphic if they exist in different morphological phases, e.g., yeast or mould, at different stages of their life cycle. Some of the systemic mycoses are dimorphic infections.

5.2 SUPERFICIAL MYCOSES
The superficial infections are common in all environments. Most are unlikely to be imported although travelling conditions in hot and humid climates may lead to the

development of tinea or dermatophytosis or *Malassezia* infections. Both are most likely to have originated from organisms already carried by the traveller but present clinically during or after exposure to a hot climatic condition. Tinea cruris (dermatophytosis of the groin) presenting in someone returning from the tropics, would be an example. Likewise tinea pedis can be exacerbated by the moist and humid conditions on the foot and can become secondarily infected with gram negative bacteria as well. There are however a few less common mycoses that can only be acquired in tropical areas.

Tinea imbricata is a form of tinea corporis which occurs in the West Pacific, Indonesia and some remote areas of Brazil and central America. It is caused by

Figure 5.1   Tinea capitis

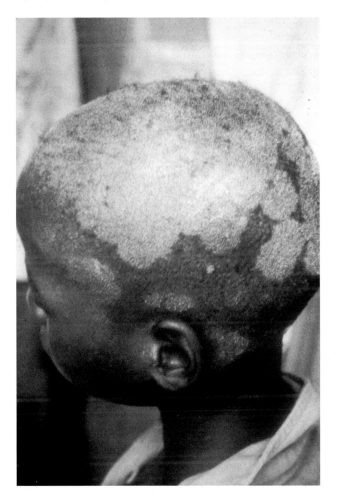

Trichophyton concentricum and is occasionally acquired by individuals working in an endemic area. It is seldom seen in short term visitors. It is clinically characteristic, presenting with concentric and often extensive concentric rings of scales on the trunk or limbs. The diagnosis is confirmed by cultural identification of the organism.

Tinea capitis due to organisms non-endemic in Europe can be imported into a city with visiting children or with immigrants. These are usually due to anthropophilic organisms transmitted from child to child and they present with scaling and hair loss (2). The organisms range from *Trichophyton violaceum* (East Africa and Indian subcontinent) to *Microsporum audouinii* (West Africa). *Trichophyton tonsurans* has become established in some European cities. Although it is also seen as an endemic infection in Europe it is likely that the recent surge in infection rates has followed an earlier increased prevalence of infections due to this organism in the USA. It is predominantly but by no means exclusively seen in children of African Caribbean origin. It remains important to identify the causes of cases of tinea capitis by microscopy and culture (figure 5.1).

Tinea nigra caused by *Phaeoanellomyces werneckii* is also occasionally seen as an imported infection. It presents as a black or brown macule, usually on the palms. There is scaling but generally this is not easy to define. It may be mistaken for an acral lentigo but skin scraping with demonstration of the presence of pigmented hyphae in direct microscopy is the best way of establishing the diagnosis. Often however these are diagnosed after a diagnostic biopsy to exclude an early acral melanoma.

Scytalidium infections due to *Scytalidium hyalinum* and *S. dimidiatum* (formerly *Hendersonula toruloidea*) which normally present as scaly dermatosis affecting the palms, soles and toe webs or onychomycosis are a mainly seen in immigrants from the tropics (3). They mimic dry type infections caused by *Trichophyton rubrum*. However occasionally they develop as nail infections in tourists who have spent weeks or months in a tropical environment. They do not respond to the antifungals that are currently available. → needs COMBINATION antifungal Rx

Tourists frequently present with pityriasis versicolor on returning from overseas travel. This is not strictly speaking an imported infection but has been acquired under the conditions prevailing in a hot sunny environment against a background of the carriage of *Malassezia globosa,* the usual cause, on peri-follicular skin (4). In a similar way *Malassezia* folliculitis is also seen in patients taking an overseas holiday when it presents with itchy follicular papules and pustules on the upper trunk or chest.

5.3 SUBCUTANEOUS MYCOSES

The subcutaneous mycoses, or mycoses of implantation, are infections caused by fungi that have been introduced directly into the dermis or subcutaneous tissue through a penetrating injury, such as a thorn prick. Although many are tropical infections, some, such as sporotrichosis, are also seen in temperate climates; any of these infections may present as an imported disease in a patient who has originated from an endemic area, sometimes many years after leaving the endemic area. The main subcutaneous mycoses are sporotrichosis, mycetoma, and chromoblastomycosis. Less frequent infections include lobomycosis and subcutaneous zygomycosis.

5.3.1 Sporotrichosis

Sporotrichosis is a subcutaneous or systemic fungal infection caused by the dimorphic fungus, *Sporothrix schenckii,* which grows on decaying vegetable matter, such as plant debris, leaves, and wood (5). The main endemic areas are North, South, and

Figure 5.2   Sporotrichosus: lymphangitic form

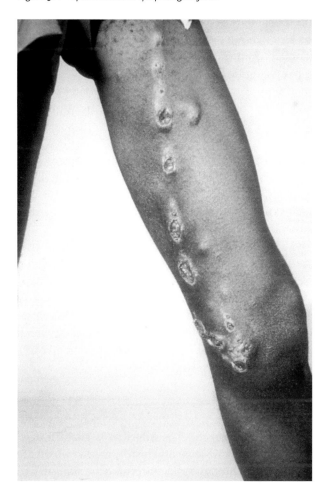

Central America (6), including the southern United States and Mexico, as well as in Africa, Egypt, Japan, and Australia. Infections are now rare in much of Europe. The most frequent site of this infection is the dermis or subcutis. The organism is introduced into the skin through a local injury. However, there is a rare systemic form of sporotrichosis whose clinical features range from pulmonary infection to arthritis or meningitis.

Subcutaneous sporotrichosis includes two main forms: lymphangitic and fixed infections. The lymphangitic form usually develops on exposed skin sites such as hands or feet (figure 5.2). The first sign of infection is the appearance of a dermal nodule that breaks down into a small ulcer. Draining lymphatics become inflamed and swollen, and a chain of secondary nodules develops along the course of the lymphatic; these may also break down and ulcerate. In the fixed variety, which accounts for about 15% of cases, the infection remains localized to a single site, such as the face, and an inflamed granulomatous lesion develops that may subsequently ulcerate.

   Fixed lesions have a granulomatous appearance and can closely mimic cutaneous leishmaniasis whereas the lymphangitic lesions can be caused by other organisms such as *Mycobacterium marinum, Nocardia* as well as some *Leishmania* spp. Sporotrichosis can occur in individuals coming to a temperate area from overseas – it is rarely seen in tourists.

The best sources of diagnostic material are smears, exudates, and biopsies. The yeasts of *S. schenckii* are scarcely distributed in lesions and very rarely seen in direct microscopic examination or histology. Culture is the best method of diagnosis and the organism can be readily isolated on Sabouraud's agar. In biopsy material yeasts may be surrounded by an eosinophilic halo or asteroid body.

The traditional treatment is a saturated solution of potassium iodide which is given in a dose of 1 ml tds and the doses increased each day very gradually until a daily dose of 4-6 ml tds is achieved (7). Potassium iodide is unpleasant to taste and can also induce salivary gland enlargement as well as nausea and vomiting. Alternative treatments include itraconazole, 200 mg daily, or terbinafine, 250 mg daily, which are better tolerated, and intravenous amphotericin B for deep infection. In all cases treatment is continued for at least 2 weeks after clinical resolution.

5.3.2 Mycetoma (maduromycosis, madura foot)

Mycetoma is a chronic localized infection caused by different species of fungi (eumycetoma) or actinomycetes (actinomycetoma) (8). The infection is characterized by the formation of visible aggregates of the causative organisms, grains, which are surrounded by abscesses. These may drain through sinus tracts onto the skin surface or invade adjacent bone. The disease progresses by direct spread. The organisms are implanted subcutaneously, usually after a penetrating injury e.g. from an implanted thorn. Infections develop very slowly and may present years after an initial, and, often unnoticed, injury. The habitat of the causative organisms are soil or plants. Mycetomas are mainly, but not exclusively, found in the dry tropics where there is low annual rainfall. They are sporadic infections that are seldom common, even in endemic areas. They are seen regularly as uncommon imported conditions in those originating from the tropics and they may present many years after the individual has left an endemic area.

Actinomycetomas due to *Nocardia* species are most common in Central America and Mexico. In other parts of the world the commonest organism is a fungus, *Madurella mycetomatis*. The actinomycete *Streptomyces somaliensis* is most often isolated from patients originating from Sudan and the Middle East.

The clinical features of both eu- and actino-mycetomas are very similar. They are most common on the foot, lower leg, or hand, although head or back involvement may also occur. Infection of the chest wall can occur with *Nocardia* infections.

The earliest stage of infection is a painless nodule that gradually enlarges with the development of draining sinus tracts over the surface (figure 5.3, 5.4). Local tissue swelling, chronic sinus formation, and later bone invasion may result in deformity.

Figure 5.3   Mycetoma on the foot

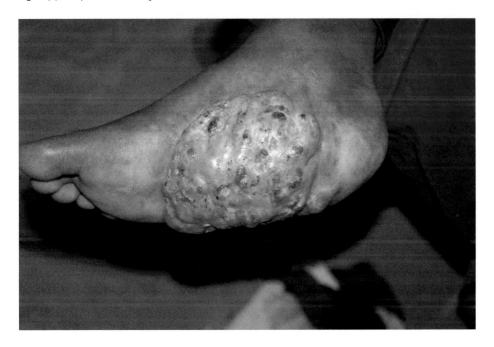

Lesions are only occasionally painful, particularly when new sinus tracts are about to penetrate to the skin surface.

The appearance of a hard subcutaneous swelling with overlying draining sinuses, and often localised overlying increased sweating, is typical although the earliest lesions without sinuses are difficult to diagnose without a biopsy. The increase in sweating may however occur in such lesions.

Actinomycosis is an endogenous infection originating in the mouth, uterus or chest and lesions with discharging sinuses, similar to the appearances of a mycetoma, are seen at such sites. Strictly speaking, though, it is not a mycetoma.

Figure 5.4   Mycetoma on the back

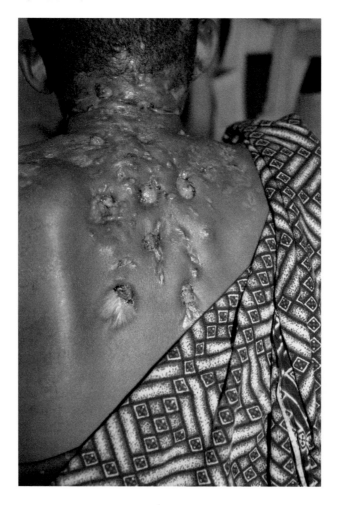

X-ray changes include periosteal thickening and proliferation as well as the development of lytic lesions in the bone. Magnetic resonance imaging is very useful in identifying the extent of bone and soft tissue lesions at an earlier stage.

Mycetoma grains may be obtained by opening a pustule or sinus tract with a sterile needle and gently squeezing the edges. Grains are 250 to 1000 μm white, black, or red particles that can be seen with the naked eye. Direct microscopic examination of grains will show whether the grain is composed of the small actinomycete or broader fungal filaments and its colour (figure 5.5). In general, it is not possible to distinguish the fine actinomycete filaments in KOH mounts or, in the case of histopathological sections, in hematoxylin/eosin-stained material. Grains (50 to 250 μm) are found within neutrophil abscesses and there are also scattered giant cells and fibrosis. The size and shape of grains visualised in histopathology may help in their identification, although with nonpigmented fungal causes of mycetoma this is seldom sufficient.

Actinomycetomas generally respond to antibiotics such as a combination of sulphamethoxazole-trimethoprim plus rifampin or dapsone and streptomycin (9). Amikacin may also be used in recalcitrant Nocardia infections. The response in all but a few cases is good.

A trial of therapy with itraconazole, terbinafine or griseofulvin is worth attempting in fungal mycetomas although responses are unpredictable; some cases of M.

Figure 5.5   Direct microscopy of grains of eumycetoma (Potassium hydroxide x 40)

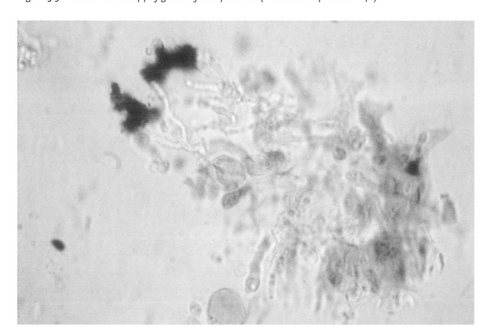

mycetomatis infection respond to ketoconazole. Radical surgery, usually amputation, is the definitive procedure and may have to be used in advanced cases.

5.3.3 Chromoblastomycosis (chromomycosis)

Chromoblastomycosis is a chronic fungal infection of the skin and subcutaneous tissues caused by pigmented or dematiaceous fungi that are implanted into the dermis from the environment (10). The infection can be caused by a number of different pigmented fungi, the commonest being *Phialophora verrucosa, Fonsecaea pedrosoi, F. compactum, Wangiella dermatitidis,* and *Cladophialophora carrionii.*

The vast majority of infections are caused by *F. pedrosoi* and *C. carrionii* which can be isolated from plant debris (11). As with other subcutaneous mycoses, infection follows implantation through a tissue injury often in agricultural workers. The infection is a sporadic condition in Central and South America, the Caribbean region, Africa, the Far East and Australia. It may occur as an imported infection outside the usual endemic areas but this is a rare occurrence.

The initial site of the infection is usually the feet, legs or arms. These early lesions are small nodules that slowly expand over months or years. Established lesions are large wart like nodules or flat atrophic plaques (figure 5.6). Individual lesions may be thick and often develop secondary bacterial infection. Spread is by direct extension over

Figure 5.6   Chromoblastomycosis on the leg

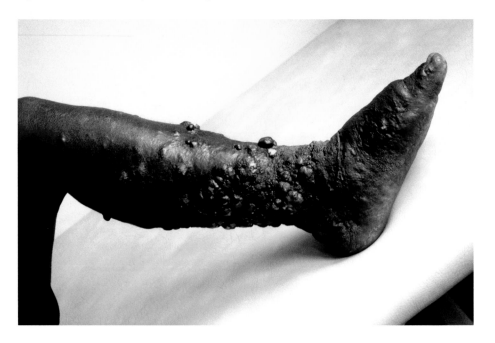

the skin. Complications of chromoblastomycosis include local lymphedema lead-ing to elephantiasis and squamous carcinomas in some chronic lesions. The early lesions can only be diagnosed by biopsy although once the warty changes have devel-oped other conditions, such as verrucous tuberculosis with more extensive lesions, have to be distinguished from mossy foot secondary to chronic lymphedema caused by lymphatic filariasias.

The typical brown sclerotic or muriform fungal cells can be seen in skin scrap-ings using KOH mounts taken from the skin surface of lesions, particularly those areas where there is a small dark spot on the affected skin surface. It is always worth scraping the surface of suspected lesions as it provides a rapid diagnosis. Histo-logy of biopsied material is also useful as the pathological changes and presence of muriform cells are both typical. The histology shows a mixed neutrophil and gra-nulomatous response with small neutrophil abscesses and pseudo-epitheliomatous hyperplasia. The organisms, which are often intracellular and clumped, have a single or double septum and thick cell wall.

The main treatments for chromoblastomycosis are itraconazole, 200 mg daily, ter-binafine, 250 mg daily (11); in extensive cases, intravenous amphotericin B (up to 1 mg/kg daily) or one of the aforementioned drugs together with flucytosine may be used. The local application of heat has been described in some instances as helpful in shrinking lesions. The responses of these fungi to different antifungals does not ap-pear to differ significantly, although there is some evidence that C. carrionii responds more rapidly to both itraconazole or terbinafine. Treatment is continued until there is clinical resolution of lesions, usually after several months of therapy.

5.3.4 Phaeohyphomycosis (phaeomycotic cyst, cystic chromomycosis)

Phaeohyphomycosis is a rare infection characterized by the formation of subcuta-neous inflammatory cysts. It is caused by dematiaceous fungi, the most common of which are Exophiala jeanselmei and Wangiella dermatitidis, but over one hundred other species have been described as causative agents (12). Although these organisms are pigmented they form short irregular pigmented hyphae in tissue. The infection may occur in any climatic area, although it is commoner in the tropics. It occurs not in-frequently as an imported infection although it is rarely recognised prior to histology of an excised lesion. It may also appear in immunosuppressed patients. The lesions present as large cysts which may be surgically removed the diagnosis becoming ap-parent after excision e.g. around the knee. They may mimic other conditions such as Baker's cysts. Histologically, the cyst wall consists of macrophages and other inflam-matory cells surrounded by a fibrous capsule, and the short fungal hyphae lie within the macrophage zone. Although the fungi in tissue lesions are usually pigmented, this is not always the case. The treatment is surgical excision without chemotherapy, although relapse can occur, particularly in immunocompromised patients.

5.3.5 Other subcutaneous infections

Subcutaneous zygomycosis occasionally presents as an imported condition. There are two forms caused respectively by *Basidiobolus ranarum* (*B. haptosporus*), and *Conidiobolus coronatus*. They present as localized hard swellings around the limb girdles in the case of the former and the central facial tissues with the latter. The organisms can be seen on biopsy and lesions usually respond to oral treatment with potassium iodide, given in similar doses to those used in sporotrichosis. Ketoconazole or itraconazole have also been used.

5.4 SYSTEMIC MYCOSES

The systemic mycoses generally invade deep structures such as the lungs, liver and spleen as well as skin and mucosal surfaces. They may spread via the blood stream to produce generalized or localised disseminated infections affecting the skin. There are two main varieties – the opportunistic and the endemic respiratory mycoses. Only the endemic mycoses are occasionally responsible for causing imported infections.

The endemic respiratory mycoses are histoplasmosis (classic and African types), blastomycosis, coccidioidomycosis, paracoccidioidomycosis, and infections due to *Penicillium marneffei*. The clinical manifestations of these infections depend on the underlying state of the patient, and follow broadly similar clinical patterns in all infections. These infections may also affect otherwise healthy individuals. They have well-defined endemic areas determined by environmental conditions. The usual route of entry in these infections is via the lung. They may be seen outside their endemic area as imported infections, although skin lesions are uncommon.

5.4.1 Histoplasmosis

In humans there are two main diseases caused, respectively, by two variants of *Histoplasma capsulatum*: *H. capsulatum* var. *capsulatum* and *H. capsulatum* var. *duboisii*. They can be distinguished because in tissue they produce yeasts of different sizes, the *capsulatum* variety producing cells from 2 to 5 µm in diameter, *duboisii* are cells of 10 to 15 µm in diameter. The other important difference is their epidemiology (13). The two types of human infections are histoplasmosis and African histoplasmosis.

The pattern of disease is illustrated best with histoplasmosis. Histoplasmosis results from infection with the dimorphic fungus *H. capsulatum* var. *capsulatum*. The infection starts as a pulmonary infection that, in most individuals, is asymptomatic and heals spontaneously, the only evidence of exposure being the development of a positive intradermal skin test reaction to histoplasmin. However, in addition, there are symptomatic and invasive forms of disease that include respiratory infections and acute or chronic pulmonary histoplasmosis as well as a disseminated infection that may spread to affect the skin and mucous membranes as well as other sites such as the adrenal. Histoplasmosis occurs in many countries from the Americas to Africa, India, and the Far East. In the United States it is endemic in the central states and around the Mississippi and Ohio River valleys, where often more than 90% of the population may have acquired the infection asymptomatically. *H. capsulatum* is an environmental saprophyte that can be isolated from soil, particularly when it is contaminated with bird or bat excreta. The disease is acquired by inhalation of spores, and epidemics of respiratory infection may occur in persons exposed to a spore laden environment when exploring caves or cleaning sites heavily contaminated with bird droppings, such as bird roosts or barns. Amongst travelers, therefore, cave explorers are often affected by acute infections. Many patients, though, have no obvious history of exposure. It also causes a rapidly progressive disseminated infection in patients with disease affecting cellular immune capacity, such as AIDS (14).

The spectrum of histoplasmosis includes asymptomatic as well as benign symptomatic infections and a progressive disseminated variety with blood stream spread to multiple organs. Skin lesions occur but are not common.

There are a number of different clinical syndromes due to *Histoplasma capsulatum*. These are described below.

Acute pulmonary histoplasmosis

In this form patients are thought to have been exposed to large quantities of spores such as may be encountered in a cave. It is seen in cavers exploring in a tropical environment. The main symptoms are cough, chest pain, and fever, often with accompanying joint pains and rash – toxic erythema, erythema multiforme, or erythema nodosum. These skin rashes are not common, occurring in fewer than 15% of patients, but they have been reported to be precipitated by antifungal treatment of the acute infection. The diagnosis is often made on the history of exposure in a suitable environment. The chest X-ray shows diffuse mottling. Serology may not become positive in the early stages of this disease.

Chronic pulmonary histoplasmosis

This usually occurs in adults and presents with pulmonary consolidation and cavitation, closely resembling tuberculosis. Skin involvement is not seen.

Disseminated histoplasmosis

In acute forms of the disease there is dissemination to other organs such as the liver and spleen, lymphoreticular system, and bone marrow. Patients present with progressive weight loss and fever. This form is the type that is most likely to occur in untreated AIDS patients, who often develop skin lesions as a manifestation of disseminated infection (15). These are papules, small nodules, or molluscum contagiosum-like lesions that may subsequently develop into shallow ulcers. Diffuse micronodular pulmonary infiltrates may also develop. Patients have progressive and severe weight loss, fever, anemia, and hepatosplenomegaly.

There are also more slowly evolving disseminated forms of histoplasmosis which may present with oral ulcers. Patients who may have left an endemic area years before, may present with an isolated lesion such as a chronic oral or laryngeal ulcer or adrenal insufficiency.

Table 5.2 Skin manifestations and imported systemic mycoses

Disease	Endemic area	Presenting skin features	Diagnosis	Treatment
blastomycosis *Blastomyces dermatitidis*	North America, Central Africa	Rare as an imported infection. Granulomatous and crusted skin lesions.	culture and histology – large yeasts which produce daughters cells on a broad base	itraconazole
coccididiodomycosis *Coccidioides immitis*	dry west coast USA, Mexico, Colombia, Venezuela, Argentina	Occasional erythema nodosum in primary infection. Ulcers, abscesses and granulomas rare. Tourists can acquire acute infections while passing through an endemic region including some common US tourist destinations.	culture, serology, histopathology – large endospore (50-100 μ) containing spherules seen in various stages of development	itraconazole, amphotericin B
paracoccidiodomycosis *Paracoccidioides brasiliensis*	Mexico, Central and South America	Ulcers and granulomas around orifices e.g. mouth, anus. Rare if ever seen in tourists. May present.	culture, serology, histopathology – characteristic multiple budding yeasts in tissue	itraconazole
infection due to *Penicillium marneffei*	Southeast Asia, Thailand, South China, Hong Kong	Multiple papules, often with central umbilication, ulcers. Risk in HIV positive travelers to endemic areas	culture, smears (bone marrow), histopathology – small yeasts with dividing septa	itraconazole

The diagnosis of histoplasmosis is established by identifying the small intracellular yeast-like cells of Histoplasma in sputum, peripheral blood, bone marrow, or in biopsy specimens. The identity of the organism should be confirmed by culture; it grows as a mould at room temperature. Serology is often useful in diagnosis. A rising complement fixation titer indicates dissemination. Precipitins detected by immuno-diffusion, are also valuable since the presence of antibodies to specific antigens, H and M antigens, correlates well with active or recent infection. A new development, particularly helpful in AIDS patients, has been serological tests for the detection of circulating Histoplasma antigens. In histopathological material, *H. capsulatum* is intracellular and is often seen in macrophages. The cells are small oval cells (2 to 4 μm in diameter) with small buds.

The choice of therapy for histoplasmosis depends on the severity of the illness. For patients with some disseminated or localized forms of the disease, oral itraconazole (200 to 400 mg daily) is highly effective. It has also been used for long-term sup-pressive treatment of the disease in AIDS patients after primary therapy either with itraconazole or amphotericin B. Intravenous amphotericin B (up to 1 mg/kg daily) is given to patients with widespread and severe infections.

Table 5.2 summarises the clinical skin lesions that may occur with the other systemic mycoses as an imported infection (16,17,18,19,20, 21).

However, the main diseases which can occur, are coccidioidomycosis which may present in travelers with erythema nodosum (18) or erythema multiforme or with disseminated ulcers of skin granulomas. It is more common for coccidioidomycosis to present with internal lesions such as lung granulomas.

Paracoccidioidomycosis is also seen rarely as an imported infection with disseminated skin lesions often around the mucocutaneous junctions e.g. mouth, or conjunctivae (figure 5.7) (19).

Penicillium marneffei infection is also regularly seen in travelers who are HIV positive, visiting endemic parts of Asia (20,21). It often presents with disseminated umbilicated skin papules on the face and trunk. The extent of these lesions is remarkable. Skin biopsy and histology plus culture are usually sufficient. It is a fallacy that these infections are difficult to diagnose although from time to time even an experienced laboratory misses the organisms.

Imported mycoses are seldom common but they are seen regularly and it is important to consider the diagnosis where possible in individuals who have visited remotes areas. As always with imported infection it is always important to take an accurate travel history so that the movements of the individual can be correlated with the potential for exposure.

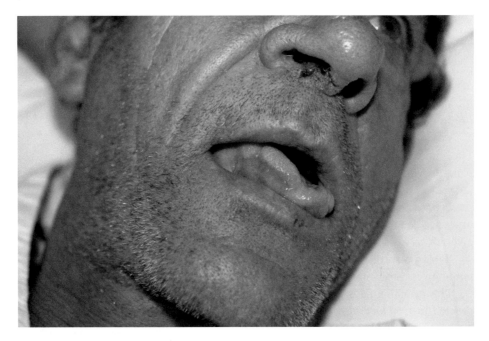

Figure 5.7   Paracoccidioidomycosis: lesions on lip and tongue

REFERENCES

1   Kibbler CC, MacKenzie DWR, Odds FC (eds.). Principles and Practice of Clinical Mycology. Chichester: Wiley, 1996.

2   Ghannoum M, Isham N, Hajjeh R, Cano M, Al-Hasawi F, Yearick D, Warner J, Long L, Jessup C, Elewski B. Tinea capitis in Cleveland: survey of elementary school students. *J Am Acad Dermatol* 2003;48:189-93.

3   Hay RJ, Moore MK. Clinical features of superficial fungal infections caused by *Hendersonula toruloidea* and *Scytalidium hyalinum*. *Br J Dermatol* 1984;110:677-83.

4   Crespo Erchiga V. Delgado Florencio V. Malassezia species in skin diseases. *Cur Op Infect Dis* 2002;15:133-42.

5   Winn RE. A contemporary view of sporotrichosis. *Curr Top Med Mycol* 1995;6:73-94.

6   Pappas PG, Tellez I, Deep AE, Nolasco D, Holgado W, Bustamante B. Sporotrichosis in Peru: description of an area of hyperendemicity. *Clin Infect Dis* 2000;30:65-70.

7   Kauffman CA. Hajjeh R. Chapman SW. Practice guidelines for the management of patients with sporotrichosis. For the Mycoses Study Group. Infectious Diseases Society of America. *Clin Infect Dis* 2000;30:684-7.

8   Hay RJ, Mahgoub ES, Leon G, al Sogair S, Welsh O. Mycetoma. *J Med Vet Mycol* 1992;30(suppl 1):41.

9   Welsh O, Saminas MC, Rodriquez MA. Treatment of eumycetoma and actino-mycetoma. *Curr Top Med Mycol* 1995;6:47-71.

10   Restrepo A. Treatment of tropical mycoses. *J Am Acad Dermatol* 1994;31:S91.

11   Esterre P. Treatment of chromomycosis with terbinafine: Preliminary results of an open pilot study. *Br J Dermatol* 1996;134(46):33.

12   Matsumoto T, Ajello L, Matsuda T, Furue M. Developments in hyalohyphomyco-sis and phaeohyphomycosis. *J Med Vet Mycol* 1994;32(1):329.

13   Cano MV, Hajjeh RA. The epidemiology of histoplasmosis: a review. *Seminars Resp Infect* 2001;16:109.

14   Wheat LJ, Slama TG, Zeekel ML. Histoplasmosis in the acquired immune defi-ciency syndrome. *Am J Med* 1985;78:203.

15   Wheat J. Endemic mycoses in AIDS: A clinical review. *Clin Microbiol Rev* 1995;8:146-59.

16   Lemos LB, Guo M, Baliga M. Blastomycosis: organ involvement and etiologic diagnosis. A review of 123 patients from Mississippi. *Annls Diagnostic Pathol* 2000;4:391.

17   Rosenstein NE, Emery KW, Werner SB, Kao A, Johnson R, Rogers D, Vugia D, Reingold A, Talbot R, Plikaytis BD, Perkins BA, Majjeh RA. Risk factors for se-vere pulmonary and disseminated coccidioidomycosis: Kern County, California, 1995-1996. *Clin Infect Dis* 2001;32:708.

18   Braverman IM. Protective effects of erythema nodosum in coccidioidomycosis. *Lancet* 1999;353:168.

19   Del Negro G, Lacaz CS, Fiorillo (eds). Paracoccidioidomicose. Sao Paulo: Sarvier Editora, 1982.

20   Chariyalertsak S, Sirisanthana T, Supparatpinyo K, Nelson KE. Seasonal vari-ation of disseminated *Penicillium marneffei* infections in northern Thailand: A clue to the reservoir? *J Infect Dis* 1996;173:1490-3.

21   Supparatpinyo K, Khamwam C, Baosoung V, Nelson KE, Sirisanthana T. Disseminated *Penicillium marneffei* infection in Southeast Asia. *Lancet* 1994;344:110-3.

6 Mycobacterial infections

W.R. Faber

6.1 INTRODUCTION

Mycobacterial infections comprise infections that are caused by the different species of the genus *Mycobacterium*. They are thin, slightly curved to straight non-motile bacilli, which can be visualized only by special staining techniques.

On the basis of clinical criteria they can be divided in three groups: (1,2)

1 includes strict pathogens for humans and animals,
2 potentially pathogenic mycobacteria,
3 normally saprophytic species that are non-pathogenic or only exceptionally pathogenic. This last group is often referred to as non-tuberculous mycobacteria (NTM), MOTT (mycobacteria other than tuberculosis), or 'atypical' mycobacteria.

Most mycobacteria give rise to localized and often harmless infections of the skin. In immune competent patients the disease is in general localized, although lymphatic spread, so-called nodular lymphangitis, is well known in for instance *M. marinum* infections.

As mycobacteria are intracellular microorganisms the immunological response of the host is an immune reaction resulting in a granulomatous tissue reaction. In immune compromised patients infections with non-tuberculous mycobacteria may lead to extensive disease. And recently it was found that patients with genetic deficiencies in cytokine type I receptors suffer from, sometimes fatal, infections by weakly pathogenic mycobacteria.

Mycobacteria responsible for most cutaneous disease are *M. marinum*, *M. ulcerans*, *M. fortuitum*, *M. chelonae* and *M. avium-intracellulare*, with exclusion of *M. leprae*. Cutaneous disease may be due to inoculation, by trauma or iatrogenic; may be contiguous with underlying osteomyelitis or lymphadenitis or may be part of disseminated disease. More rarely infections are caused by *M. szulgai*, *M. kansasii* and *M. haemophilum* (1,2,3).

Leprosy, which dates back to approximately 600 BC in India, has still a new case detection rate between 600 000 and 700 000 yearly. Leprosy with its sometimes devastating consequences will be addressed in chapter 7. Buruli ulcer, named after the area in Uganda where prevalence was high, has spread to new areas, especially in Africa, and is addressed in chapter 9.

6.2 TUBERCULOSIS

6.2.1 Introduction
The range of clinical manifestations of cutaneous tuberculosis provides a classical example of the varying immune response of the host towards the infection with mycobacteria, which also depends on previous exposure to other mycobacteria and the route of infection (4,5).

Cutaneous tuberculosis has nowadays become a rare disease in inhabitants of the Western World. Therefore, the majority of cutaneous tuberculosis cases will be diagnosed in immigrants.

6.2.2 Epidemiology
Cutaneous tuberculosis was diagnosed in 2 to 4% of outpatients in dermatological clinics in Great Britain at the beginning of the 20th century. The same figures have been reported in studies from Asia in the middle of the last century and appear there to be decreasing.

In the majority the initial (primary) infection is by inhalation of infected droplets from patients with active pulmonary disease. In circumstances where *M. tuberculosis* is common as in Third World countries as well as in some medical settings in the Western World infection by inoculation of the skin can occur.

6.2.3 Clinical picture
Cutaneous tuberculosis can be classified according to four categories (see table 6.1):
I   Primary infection (in tuberculin negative persons).
II Secondary infection (in tuberculin positive persons):
   A   exogenous inoculation,
   B   endogenous inoculation by contiguous spread,
   C   endogenous inoculation by haematogenous route.
III Bacille Calmette-Guérin (BCG) infection.
IV Immunological reactions ('tuberculids').

Primary infection = tuberculous chancre
Due to exogenous inoculation of *M. tuberculosis*. It accounts for 2% of all cases of cutaneous tuberculosis. The lesion starts, 2 to 4 weeks after inoculation, with a smooth

papule or nodule which enlarges in the course of several weeks to a plaque which ulcerates. The ulcer has undermined edges, and is painless. After 3 to 8 weeks non-tender regional lymphadenopathy develops which may suppurate to form a 'cold' abscess which then may spontaneously drain with sinus tract formation. This process in general heals spontaneously with atrophic scarring in 3 to 12 months. Primary lesions are mainly localised on the face and extremities of children, but inoculation by instrumentation, such as injections and surgical procedures, is possible. It may evolve in some cases into scrofuloderma, lupus vulgaris, or verrucous lesions.

Differential diagnosis: other causes of ulceration, and chronic infections such as subcutaneous mycoses, cutaneous leishmaniasis, and malignant tumours.

Table 6.1   Classification of cutaneous tuberculosis

I	Primary infection	tuberculous chancre
II	Secondary infection	
	A. exogenous	warty tuberculosis
	B. endogenous	• contiguous spread: scrofuloderma • autoinoculation: orificial tuberculosis

	C. hematogenous	• chronic:
		    - lupus vulgaris
		    - tuberculous gumma
		• acute:
		    - acute miliary tuberculosis

III	BCG infections	
IV	Immunologic reaction to tuberculosis elsewhere: tuberculids	• tuberculonecrotic tuberculid • lichen scrofulosorum • erythema induration of Bazin • erythema nodosum

Adapted from ref. 4

Secondary infection
Secondary infection comprises the great majority of all cases of cutaneous tuberculosis.

Warty tuberculosis = tuberculosis verrucosa cutis
Due to exogenous inoculation of *M. tuberculosis* in the skin of a person with an acquired immune response towards *M. tuberculosis*. Therefore, due to the rapid cell mediated response the infection stays localised, and regional lymphadenopathy is not prominent. It is reported to be the most common form of cutaneous tuberculosis in Asia.

The lesion develops from an asymptomatic reddish-brown papule into a verrucous plaque of varying shape and size. The surface is hyperkeratotic and rough to verrucous (wartlike) with deep fissures. The lesion can be moist from serous exudates to purulent due to secondary bacterial infection. The plaque may heal spontaneously in the course of months to years, with atrophic scarring in one place and extension in the other. Lesions are mostly localised on the limbs and buttocks of children in endemic areas. It is an occupational risk for workers in several professions such as pathologists (so called prosectors wart), butchers and abattoir workers. In these cases disease is mostly localised on the fingers or dorsum of the hands.

Differential diagnosis: common wart in the initial stage. Verrucous lesion caused by atypical mycobacteria, some forms of deep mycoses as blastomycosis and chromomycosis, some forms of South American leishmaniasis, verrucous tertiary syphilis and skin cancer.

Scrofuloderma = tuberculosis cutis colliquativa

Due to contiguous spread from a deeper localised infection such as lymph node or in some cases bone. Initially there is an indurated inflammatory area overlying the deeper infection. Due to suppuration fluctuating nodules develop, which ulcerate with the formation of sinus tracks. In the course of time cordlike scars or keloids develop. The lesions heal in the course of years with characteristic pattern of fibrosis and scarring. Recurrence of drainage is common. The lesions are mostly localised over the lymph glands in the neck.

Differential diagnosis: deep mycoses as sporotrichosis and coccidioidiomycosis, actinomycosis, hidradenitis suppurativa in axillary lesions, lymphogranuloma venerum in inguinal lesions, chronic bacterial osteomyelitis when localised over bone.

Orifical tuberculosis = tuberculosis ulcerosa cutis et mucosae

Due to autoinoculation of organisms from an active infection at a deeper site. It occurs in patients with extensive disease in who the immune reaction is suppressed, and therefore bears a poor diagnosis. It is reported to be quite rare. Lesions start with single or multiple nodules, which become fluctuant and ulcerate with the formation of draining sinuses. The lesions are painful. Localisations are, as the name implies, characteristically around the anus, mouth, nose and genitalia, in patients with advanced disease.

Differential diagnosis: other diseases with ulcerations as aphtous ulcers, herpes simplex lesions, ulcerations of venereal diseases.

Lupus vulgaris

Due to reactivation in patients with a high degree of immunity after earlier haematogenous dissemination. However, lupus vulgaris lesions have also been described in warty tuberculosis, scrofuloderma, and after Bacille Calmette-Guérin (BCG) inoculation. It was the most common manifestation of cutaneous tuberculosis in Europe. But the incidence has dropped sharply after World ward II. It is common in developing countries.

The lesions start with brown-red papules which in the classical form extend to plaques with peripheral activity with an irregular border and central healing with atrophic scar formation with depigmentation (figure 6.1). The clinical picture can be very variable; besides the plaque form there is a hypertrophic form with nodules which may form a hyperkeratotic mass. The most destructive type: the ulcerative form which may erode cartilage and bone, and results in extensive scarring and even deformities. It follows a chronic course, and lesions may persist for decades, with gradual extension with progressive scarring, deformity and loss of function. The most common localisation is the face, with the nose, cheeks, mouth and earlobes

Figure 6.1   Lupus vulgaris

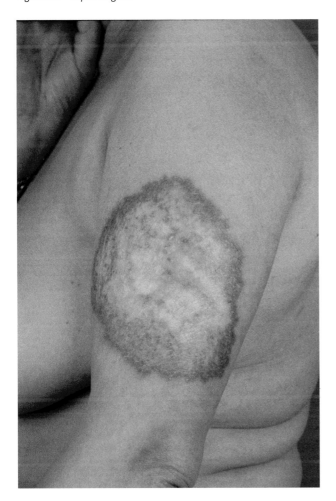

as preferential sites. In Asia and Africa lesions on legs and buttocks are common. Spinocellular carcinoma can develop in chronic lupus vulgaris lesions.

Differential diagnosis: lupoid variant of cutaneous leishmaniasis, subcutaneous mycoses, sarcoidosis, chronic discoid lupus erythematosus and basal cell carcinoma.

Tuberculous gumma = metastatic tuberculous ulcer

Due to haematogenous dissemination from a primary focus, during periods of lowered resistance with bacillaemia.

The lesion starts with a subcutaneous nodule or a fluctuant swelling. The overlying skin breaks down, resulting in an undermined ulcer with sinus formation. It then resembles scrofuloderma.

Differential diagnosis: tertiary syphilitic gumma, subcutaneous mycoses and cutaneous leishmaniasis.

Acute military tuberculosis = tuberculosis cutis miliaris disseminata

Due to extensive dissemination of *M. tuberculosis* to skin and other organs in case of complete failure of cell mediated immune reactivity. It is usually in the form of a generalized eruption of purplish papules, with vesicles on top which may break resulting in crust formation, and nodules with necrosis and ulceration. The lesions are disseminated over the whole skin with a predilection for the trunk. Due to the absence of cell mediated immune reactivity the histopathological picture is a non-specific inflammation with numerous acid fast bacilli.

Differential diagnosis: the rash is not specific and should be differentiated from other maculopapular and acneiform eruptions. The patient, however, is systemically ill, and this should be an additional clue.

BCG infections

BCG vaccination, with an attenuated strain of *M. bovis*, is practised in many areas of the world. The vaccination provokes an immune reaction which is clinically seen as an infiltrative papule which develops in 10 to 14 days at the inoculation site. It enlarges into an ulcerative lesion of approximately 1 cm at 10 to 12 weeks. It heals with scarring. After approximately 3 months the tuberculin skin test reverses from negative to positive. Complications, although infrequently, may occur in the form of progressive ulcerative infection, abscess formation, regional lymphadenitis (sometimes with scrofuloderma), lupus vulgaris and tuberculids.

Differential diagnosis: depends on the clinical picture of the complication.

Immunological reactions to tuberculosis elsewhere = tuberculids

Tuberculids are a number of dermatological manifestations, especially associated with infection with. M. *tuberculosis*. They are supposed to be due to the dissemination of M. *tuberculosis* or antigenic particles to the skin in persons with a well-established immune response. The lesions are usually widespread and symmetrical.

Agreement about the range of tuberculids was hampered by the fact that in general M. *tuberculosis* cannot be demonstrated by special stains in a biopsy, nor can it be cultured from a biopsy, and that evidence for active infection elsewhere in the body is lacking. The following are nowadays accepted to be true tuberculids.

Tuberculonecrotic tuberculid

Is the most common tuberculid nowadays. The clinical picture is that of scattered symmetric, red papules or papulopustules that become reactive with a black scab. They may heal with antituberculous treatment, but may also resolve spontaneously with a depressed scar with a hyperpigmented border.

The presence of M. *tuberculosis* DNA by means of PCR in lesions of tuberculo-necrotic tuberculid supports the tuberculous origin.

Differential diagnosis: prurigo papules, folliculitis, papular lesions of syphilis. Necrotic lesions should be differentiated from pityriasis lichenoides acuta, necrotizing vasculitis, necrotic insect bite reactions.

Lichen scrofulosorum

Is nowadays a rare manifestation of the tuberculids. Clinically it is an eruption of small lichenoid papules with a rough surface, often localised perifollicularly and grouped in nummular lichenoid plaques. PCR has also demonstrated the presence of M. *tuberculosis* DNA in lesions of lichen scrofulosorum.

Differential diagnosis: lichenoid eruptions as lichen planus, secondary syphilis, pityriasis lichenoides chronica, lichenoid drug eruptions. Due to the perifollicular distribution it has to be differentiated from keratosis follicularis, lichen nitidus, and pityriasis.

Differentiation from the micronodular form of sarcoidosis may be difficult.

Nodular vasculitis (= erythema induratum of Bazin)

Erythema induratum, described by Bazin in 1855, has been considered to be associated with tuberculosis. Nowadays it is accepted that it can be induced by numerous triggers including tuberculosis. The clinical picture is that of firm, deep, violaceous nodules and plaques on the back of the lower legs especially in middle aged women. The histopathological picture is a nodular vasculitis. M. *tuberculosis* DNA has been demonstrated in biopsies from nodular vasculitis (6).

Differential diagnosis: erythema nodosum, panniculitis, polyarteritis nodosa.

Erythema nodosum

Was in the past frequently associated with tuberculosis, but nowadays in the Western World, it is most frequently caused by streptococcal disease, sarcoidosis, drug reactions and inflammatory bowel disease, but tuberculosis still should be considered in developing countries.

Clinically it manifests itself as painful erythematous nodules on the lower legs, especially the extensor aspect. The histopathological picture is a panniculitis with vessel involvement, and gives no information on the cause.

Differential diagnosis: panniculitis, polyarteritis nodosa, erythema induratum, nodular lymphangitis.

6.2.4 Treatment

Treatment of cutaneous tuberculosis is commonly with a multiple drug regimen consisting of isoniazid, ethambutol, pyrazinamide and rifampicin.

Figure 6.2   Mycobacterium marinum infection of the finger

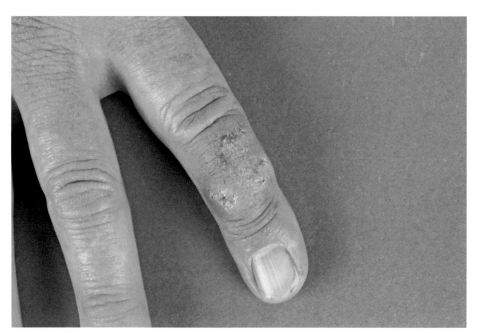

6.3 MYCOBACTERIUM MARINUM INFECTION (SWIMMING POOL GRANULOMA) (2,7,8,9)

6.3.1 Introduction
Swimming pool granuloma is caused by *Mycobacterium marinum,* a mycobacterium belonging to the atypical mycobacteria, which causes disease in fresh- and salt water fish, and occasionally in humans.

6.3.2 Epidemiology
As initial reports of cutaneous disease by *M. marinum* were associated with swimming pools, it was called swimming pool granuloma. Infection in swimming pools nowadays is rare due to proper chlorination. The distribution is world wide, occurring in fresh-brackish as well as salt water, and is prevalent in heated water (for instance in tropical aquaria) in temperate climates, and in pools and the sea in more tropical climates. In principle any water-related activity carries a potential risk for infection. Infection takes place through, in general superficially, traumatised skin.

6.3.3 Clinical picture
After a relatively long incubation period of 2 to 6 weeks the initial lesions starts as an inflammatory papule. As infection is preceded by trauma, lesions are usually localised on the back of fingers (figure 6.2) or hand, or around the knee. The papule then gradually enlarges in violaceous nodules or plaques which may ulcerate or develop a warty surface. As these lesions are painless and enlarge slowly, there is generally a delay of months to even years before a doctor's opinion is sought. These lesions may heal spontaneously; however, this may take months to years. Deep infections such as tenosynovitis, osteomyelitis, arthritis and bursitis occur infrequently. *M. marinum* infections are one of the causes of nodular lymphangitis (also called sporotrichoid spread after the lymphatic spread of sporotrichosis). Clinically, it shows nodules and/ or ulcerating lesions resulting from spread along the lymphatic vessels. Deep infections and nodular lymphangitis do not heal spontaneously.

6.3.4 Diagnosis
The clinical picture, the preferential localisation in combination with a history of aquatic activity with skin trauma, should lead to a high index of suspicion. The clinical diagnosis should be confirmed by diagnostic tests. Histopathological examination of a skin biopsy can be non-specific in the early stage of the disease. After 6 months a granulomatous reaction develops. The presence of acid-fast bacilli by special staining techniques is reported in varying percentage of cases; absence does not rule out *M. marinum* infection. Cultures can be performed from aspirates or biopsies. The optimal growth is at 30 to 32 C, and cultures should be maintained for

6 weeks. Nowadays PCR techniques from biopsy material provide the possibility of a diagnosis within days.

6.3.5 Treatment

Several treatment options exist. Treatment regimens consist of combinations containing clarithromycin, rifampicin or ethambutol. More recently the new macrolides such as clarithromycin, may be used as single drug therapy. However, no randomised studies have been performed. Response to treatment is slow, and therapy is continued to clinical cure.

6.4 MYCOBACTERIUM KANSASII INFECTIONS (2,3,10)

6.4.1 Epidemiology

M. kansasii causes diseases in humans throughout the world. It has been isolated from cattle and swine. However, water is most likely its true natural habitat. It can affect patients of all ages.

6.4.2 Clinical picture

The most common manifestation is chronic pulmonary disease. Inoculation of the skin is in general through a small wound. Cutaneous lesions are diverse: resembling pyogenic abscess, cellulitis or sporotrichosis. Cervical lymphadenitis was reported predominantly in children.

6.5 MYCOBACTERIUM SCROFULACEUM INFECTIONS (2,3,10)

6.5.1 Epidemiology

M. scrofulaceum is widely distributed, and can be isolated from tap water and soil.

6.5.2 Clinical picture

The most common infection is pulmonary. Cutaneous infection has been described as cutaneous abscesses, and sporotrichoid infection of the arms. The most common manifestation is cervical lymphadenitis in children.

6.6 MYCOBACTERIUM HEMOPHILUM INFECTIONS (2,10)

6.6.1 Epidemiology

Infections with *M. hemophilum* have been reported in a broad geographical range. The natural habitat and route of infection are unknown.

6.6.2 Clinical picture

It appears that pre- or early adolescents of both sexes are more susceptible to a mild and limited form of skin infection. It also causes cases of submandibular lymphadenitis in children.

6.7 MYCOBACTERIUM FORTUITUM INFECTIONS (2,10,11)

6.7.1 Epidemiology

M. fortuitum has been isolated from water, soil and dust. Primary cutaneous disease is seen at all ages. It has been implicated in outbreaks of hospital infections.

6.7.2 Clinical picture

The clinical manifestations are localised cases of cellulitis, frequently with draining abscesses or nodules. A history of a penetrating injury with possible soil or water contamination is often reported. Postoperative infections, in general, develop 3 weeks to 3 months after surgery. *M. fortuitum* infections can be treated by monotherapy or combination therapy with for instance, ciprofloxacin, amikacin, and clarithromycin.

6.8 MYCOBACTERIUM CHELONAE-ABSCESSUS INFECTIONS (2,11)

6.8.1 Epidemiology

Subspecies *chelonae* is common in Europe; subspecies *abscessus* is common in Africa and the United States.

6.8.2 Clinical picture

The clinical manifestations are similar as those due to *M. fortuitum*: localised cellulitis, draining abscesses or nodules. It may occur at all ages, typically after trauma or a surgical incision.

6.8.3 Treatment

Treatment of localized disease is by clarithromycin.

6.9 MYCOBACTERIUM SZULGAI INFECTIONS (2,10)

6.9.1 Epidemiology

The natural habitat of *M. szulgai* is not known. It has, however, been isolated from snails and tropical fish.

6.9.2 **Clinical picture**

The predominant localisation of infections is pulmonary. Cases of skin infection have been reported.

6.10 **MYCOBACTERIUM AVIUM-INTRACELLULARE INFECTIONS (2,3,10)**

6.10.1 **Epidemiology**

This mycobacterial species, with over 20 subtypes, occurs world wide in nature. And it may be isolated in more than 30% of faecal samples of humans.

6.10.2 **Clinical picture**

Pulmonary infection is the most common clinical manifestation. Skin involvement occurs in the course of dissemination of the pulmonary disease as papules, nodules and ulcers, and more rarely by inoculation.

6.11 **TREATMENT OF CUTANEOUS INFECTIONS BY ATYPICAL MYCOBACTERIA IN GENERAL**

Treatment of cutaneous infections by atypical mycobacteria is preferably by selecting the drugs based on the antimicrobial susceptibility profile. Empiric therapy should be started until the results of susceptibility testing are available. Empiric therapy is

Figure 6.3 Undefined atypical mycobacterial infection

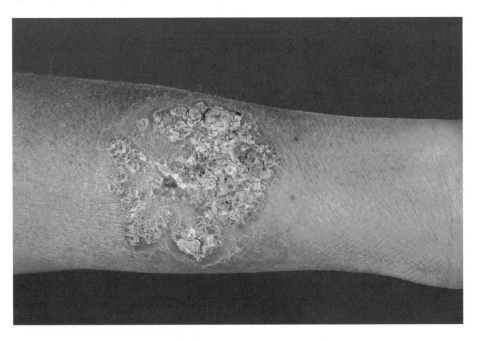

also necessary in cases of negative culture but identification by means of PCR technique. It may also be required when there are negative diagnostic tests with a clinical suspicion of mycobacterial disease; the response to treatment is then a confirmation of the clinical diagnosis (figure 6.3). Duration of treatment is not fixed, and is based on clinical judgement. It will require in general 2 to 6 months (2,3,11).

6.12 **GENERAL COMMENTS**

Although the classification of cutaneous tuberculosis has been applied to infection with *M. tuberculosis* one has to realize that in studies on cutaneous tuberculosis di-

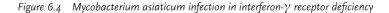

Figure 6.4   Mycobacterium asiaticum infection in interferon-γ receptor deficiency

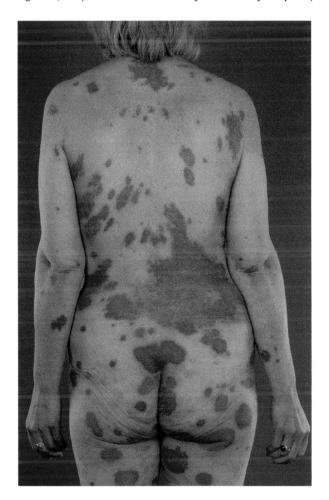

agnosis is often made on clinical and/or histopathological grounds, in part supplemented with cultures.

However, recently clinical manifestations as described for cutaneous tuberculosis have been reported for non-tuberculous mycobacteria such as lichen scrofulosorum by *M. avium,* lupus vulgaris by *M. xenopi,* papulonecrotic tuberculid reaction by *M. kansasii,* and scrofuloderma by *M. hemophilum.* In these more recent cases the infectious organism was identified by culture or PCR (12). It is, therefore, conceivable that, by application of modern molecular biological techniques on biopsies and cultures, clinical pathology which formerly would be classified as being caused by *M. tuberculosis* in fact may be caused by other (non-tuberculous) mycobacteria.

As the clinical picture of mycobacterial infection of the skin can be non-specific, a high index of suspicion is warranted. In cases of persistent infiltrative lesions or a non-healing ulcer investigation for mycobacteria is indicated. As is illustrated by the non-healing ulcer in a patient which developed during a travel in Mexico, and from whom *M. immunogenum* was cultured.

6.13 CUTANEOUS MYCOBACTERIAL INFECTIONS AND IMMUNE SUPPRESSION

Coincident with the HIV epidemic the number of infections of the skin with mycobacteria, in particular *Mycobacterium avium* complex, has increased. In patients with HIV and other forms of immune suppression lesions can present as non-healing nodules, plaques or ulceration. Depending on the degree of immune suppression widespread skin involvement may occur presenting as papules, nodules, plaques, with possible abscess formation, and ulcers. Lymph node infection can occur.

Moreover, it has been found that patients with interferon-γ and IL-12 receptor deficiencies are prone to infection with normally non-pathogenic mycobacteria. As the interferon-γ and IL-12 pathways are crucial in the development of immune response to intracellular micro-organisms, wide spread cutaneous involvement can be found (figure 6.4) (13).

REFERENCES

1 Portaels F. Epidemiology of mycobacterial diseases. *Clin Dermatol* 1995;13:207-22.
2 Hautmann G, Katsambas A, Lotti T. Non-tuberculous mycobacterial skin infections. *J Eur Acad Dermatol Venereol* 1997;9:1-35.
3 Woods GL, Washington JA. Mycobacteria other than *Mycobacterium tuberculosis:* Review of microbiologic and clinical aspects. *Rev Inf Dis* 1987;9:275-94.
4 MacGregor RR. Cutaneous tuberculosis. *Clin Dermatol* 1995;13:245-55.
5 Barbagallo J, Tager P, Ingleton R, Hirsch RJ, Weinberg JM. Cutaneous tuberculosis. Diagnosis and Treatment. *Am J Clin Dermatol* 2002;3:319-28.

6   Bayer-Gardner IB, Cox MD, Scott MA, Smoller BR. Mycobacteria other than *My-cobacterium tuberculosis* are not present in erythema induratum/nodular vasculitis: a case series and literature review of the clinical and histologic findings, *J Cutan Pathol* 2005;320:220-6.

7   Gluckman SJ. *Mycobacterium marinum. Clin Dermatol* 1995;13:273-6.

8   Jernigan JA, Farr BM. Incubation period and sources of exposure for cutaneous *Mycobacterium marinum* infection: Case report and review of the literature. *Clin Inf Dis* 2000;31:439-43.

9   Lewis FMT, Marsh BJ, Reyn CF von. Fish tanks exposure and cutaneous infections due to *Mycobacterium Marinum*: Tuberculin skin testing, treatment, and prevention. *Clin Inf Dis* 2003;37:390-7.

10 Wayne LG, Sramek HA. Agents of newly recognized or infrequently encountered mycobacterial diseases. *Clin Microbiol Rev* 1992;5:1-25.

11 Brown-Elliot BA, Wallace RJ. Clinical and taxonomic status of pathogenic non-pigmented rapidly graving mycobacteria. *Clin Microbiol Rev* 2002;15:716-46.

12 Chemlal K, Portaels F. Molecular diagnosis of nontuberculous mycobacteria. *Curr Opin Inf Dis* 2003;16:77-83.

13 Ottenhoff TH, Verreck FA, Lichtenauer-Kaligis Eg, Hoeve MA, Sanal O, van Dissel JT. Genetics, cytokines and human infectious disease: lessons from weakly pathogenic mycobacteria and salmonellae. *Nat Genet* 2002;32:97-105.

7 Leprosy

B. Naafs and W.R. Faber

7.1 INTRODUCTION

The WHO with the slogan 'elimination of leprosy by the year 2000' has induced the general belief that leprosy is irradicated. Nothing is less true. In the year 2002 more leprosy patients were diagnosed than in any year in the past. Leprosy has merely been eliminated from the statistics. This was done by changing definitions and by shortening the treatment. It is still a disease to reckon with, a disease that may lead to severe disabilities when not diagnosed in time and not treated properly (1). Doctors' delay is a big problem in Europe and the United States (2). Moreover leprosy has become one of the immune reconstitution inflammatory syndromes (IRIS), indicating that there may be a pool of *Mycobacterium leprae (M. leprae)* of unknown size (3).

In anyone who was born or has lived in a leprosy endemic area, leprosy must be suspected when a hypopigmented macule, or skin coloured, slightly erythematous or livid nodules is seen, or when a patient presents with unexplained sensory loss or muscle weakness.

Leprosy is only occasionally encountered in a tourist.

7.2 EPIDEMIOLOGY

Leprosy is still endemic in Middle and South America, in Africa south of the Sahara and in Asia from Iran to Indonesia, on some islands in the Pacific and in the Northern Territory of Australia. More than 85% of the leprosy patients live in the following countries: India, Brasil, Indonesia, Nepal, Mozambique, Madagascar, United Republic of Tanzania, Democratic Republic of the Congo and Centrale Afrique.

Leprosy is an infectious disease caused by an intracellular acid-fast bacterium: *M. leprae*. In 1873, Armauer Hansen was the first to describe the bacterium as the cause of leprosy. However the trias of Koch is still not fulfilled. It has not yet been possible to infect someone wilfully with *M. leprae*, although anecdotal reports show infection after tattooing and following the skinning and cleaning of infected armadillos for the cooking pot.

It is generally considered to be an airborne infection, directly from the oro-nasal-pharyngeal mucosa to oro-nasal-pharyngeal mucosa, but there are indications that the indirect way of infection through the soil and inoculation in the skin cannot be excluded. Even direct skin to skin contact and sexual intercourse may contribute.

It may be theorised that differences between the immune responses elicited by different routes of infection and inoculum size, skin versus nasal mucosa and possibly nerve, are responsible for the outcome of the infection. Entrance through the skin may lead to a delayed type of hypersensitivity reaction or to resistance, while through the mucous membranes it may lead to tolerance. Balance between those two routes of infection may determine the spectrum.

However, data to date suggest that the response is also modulated by genetic factors, among which HLA-DR, NRAMP-1 and small genetic differences in other membrane receptors like IL-2, IFN-gamma, Toll-like receptor and by small differences in the molecular structure of cytokines. But even more important are previous encounters with other micro-organisms and autoantigens with antigenic determinants similar to those of *M. leprae*. The final result, resistance, delayed type of hypersensitivity, tolerance, disease or no disease, tuberculoid, borderline or lepromatous leprosy with or without reactions is most likely mediated by the orchestration of the cyto- and chemokines induced in harmony with the cellular response (4).

Figure 7.1   The leprosy spectrum

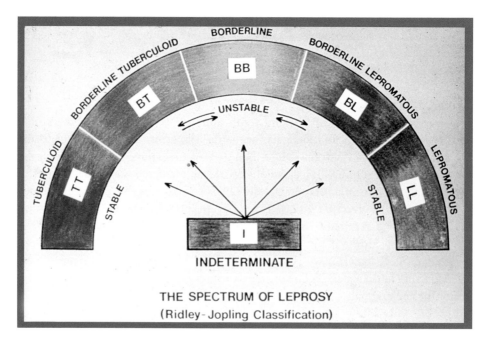

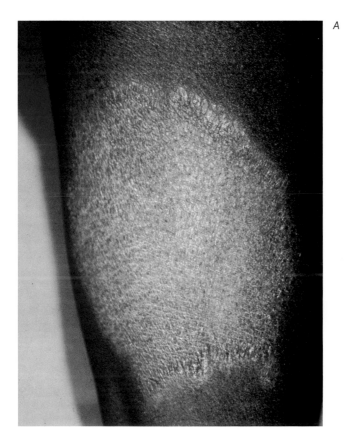

Figure 7.2   TT leprosy A: a single well-defined patch.

7.3 CLINICAL SPECTRUM

The clinical manifestations of leprosy are various, but it has been possible to classify the patients along a clinical spectrum. This was most neatly done coincidentally, but independently by Ridley and Jopling in the U.K. (5) and by Leiker in the Netherlands in 1966 (6). The classification is based on the Cell Mediated Immune response (CMI) of the patients against *M. leprae* leading to a clinical spectrum (figure 7.1).

On one side of the spectrum, with a relatively high CMI towards antigenic determinants of *M. leprae*, the tuberculoid (TT) patients are classified. They manifest clinically with one or a few well-defined hypopigmented or erythematous patches, usually with central healing and marked loss of sensation in the patch, sometimes with an enlarged peripheral nerve (figure 7.2 A,B). *M. leprae* is not detectable.

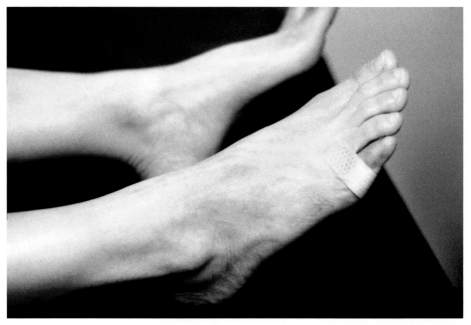

B

Figure 7.2   TT leprosy B: pure neural TT with a single enlarged cutaneous branch of the N. suralis

On the other side of the spectrum, the lepromatous patients do not develop CMI against the organism. These patients are actually teeming with bacteria; they present the perfect culture medium. The bacteria may be present anywhere in the body with the central nervous system (CNS) as a possible exception. The patients may show minimal hypopigmented or erythematous patches, ill defined and usually with the sensation still present. However, they may show glove and stocking anaesthesia with symmetrically enlarged peripheral nerves. They also may show nodules and plaques, skin coloured, erythematous, hyperpigmented or livid or, show only a diffuse infiltration (figure 7.3).

There may be loss of eyebrows (madurosis) and a more or less generalised diminished sweating. Between these two poles of the spectrum, the borderline leprosy group is found, encompassing most of the patients. The clinical range is from borderline tuberculoid (BT) leprosy with a few asymmetrical distributed well-defined tuberculoid patches and a few enlarged nerves, to borderline lepromatous (BL) leprosy with more symmetrically distributed hypopigmented or erythematous macules and/or papules and nodules. The latter are mainly located on the colder parts of the body. In the middle of the spectrum is a very unstable group, mid-borderline (BB) leprosy having lesions with an immune area (the centre of the lesion is not involved) and with typical dome-shaped elevated small plaques.

In the borderline range, patients may up- or downgrade (c.q. change their classification within the spectrum). Upgrading indicates that the patient develops more tuberculoid features, downgrading more lepromatous. In upgrading leprosy the bacterial load diminishes and in downgrading the bacteria multiplie. In a downgraded patient, a few patches may show loss of sensation whereas the other newer lesions do not or less. In an upgrading patient new tuberculoid lesions, with loss of sensation, may appear or lesions may become atrophic (heal).

Figure 7.3   LL leprosy, diffuse infiltrated; also called 'lepra bonita'

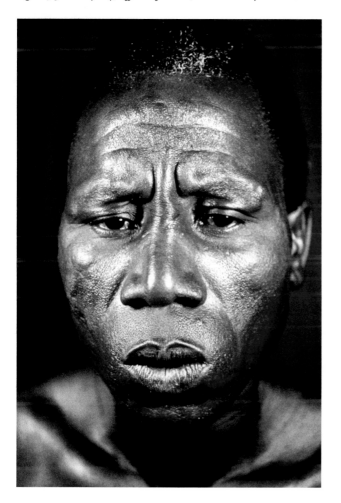

Up- and downgrading occurs either unnoticed or is accompanied by a reactional phenomenon called Type-I leprosy reaction or Reversal Reaction (RR), in which an enhanced CMI toward *M.leprae* antigenic determinants may cause irreversible nerve damage.

Indeterminate leprosy comprises a special group of leprosy patients having one or two slightly hypopigmented or erythematous macules with or without detectable loss of sensation or loss of sweating. The biopsy may show a single bacterium or a minimal lymphocytic infiltration in a dermal nerve. The diagnosis is difficult to establish and some leprologists consider it to be an early, transient form of either MB or PB leprosy, which either may heal (over 80%) or become frank MB or PB leprosy.

For operational purposes the leprosy spectrum is simplified to paucibacillary (PB) and multibacillary (MB) leprosy. PB leprosy patients are Indeterminate, TT and BT leprosy without *M. leprae* in skin smear or biopsy. MB patients are BT, BB, BL and LL patients with *M. leprae* in smear or biopsy. However in many control programs the smear services are unreliable, therefore these programs have to resort to very simple clinical criteria, some classify all patients with 5 or less lesions paucibacillary (WHO), others those with 3 or fewer lesions. The remaining patients are then classified MB (7,8).

Leprosy in children may be present as early as 3 months after birth. Usually, depending on the endemicity of leprosy and socioeconomic circumstances, leprosy manifests itself after the age of 6 years. An important reason for this is that the incubation time appears to be between 2 and 5 years. Most children, when diagnosed early, show indeterminate leprosy or leprosy with borderline features, mostly tuberculoid. Since PB leprosy needs only a few bacteria to show clinical symptoms, the clinical manifestations of tuberculoid leprosy develop earlier in life than those of lepromatous leprosy. Lepromatous leprosy, when it develops in children, seems especially confined to the head and the extremities, i.e. the colder parts of the body.

7.4 DIAGNOSIS AND CLASSIFICATION

Awareness is the most important factor for the diagnosis of leprosy. When a patient lives or has lived in a leprosy endemic country, leprosy must always be considered in the differential diagnosis of a hypopigmented or erythematous patch or a papular or nodular eruption. The same certainly applies for each condition accompanied by peripheral nerve function impairment. Hypopigmented or erythematous patches are frequently seen. An important feature of a leprosy lesion is that it does not itch but shows loss of sensation to fine touch. This can be tested by means of a piece of cottonwool made to a fine thread (figure 7.4).

The skin should not be stroked but touched with the cotton wisp. The sensation in the patch is then compared with the sensation of the surrounding normal skin by asking the patient to point where the skin was touched. It is remarkable how sensitive this investigation is. Established loss of sensation makes the diagnosis 'leprosy' very likely, especially when an enlarged nerve can be palpated. It may not be possible to test the sensation in very young children. The absence of sweat in a skin lesion after 'running', sun bathing or exposure to heat may then be a helpful diagnostic tool.

One should be aware that in the face, where hypopigmentation frequently occurs especially in children, loss of sensation occurs late, if it occurs at all. Often, patches of pityriasis alba are present in the face. These can be differentiated from leprosy by carefully describing the size and place of each lesion, and requesting that the child be brought back in 3 months time. By then a pityriasis alba spot has most likely disap-

Figure 7.4   Loss of sensation. Test with cottonwool.

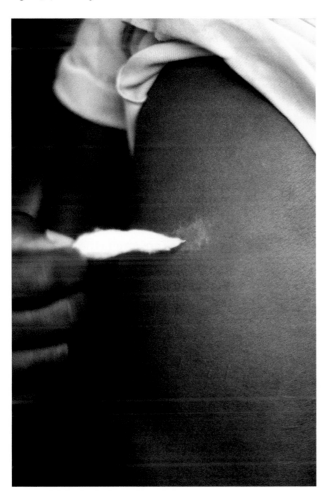

peared or changed place. A leprosy patch will remain in exactly the same spot and may have enlarged. However, the evolution of leprosy at this stage is usually slow. Be alert for a hypopigmented patch, which suddenly becomes inflamed. This is a sign of danger: a reaction may be imminent! A RR in the face often leads to facial palsy with lagophthalmus and loss of corneal sensation. This may result in blindness.

Nerves that can be inspected and palpated are the cutaneous nerves in the immediate vicinity of a patch: the great auricular, the ulnar, the median, the radiocutaneous, the lateral popliteal and the tibial posterior nerves. Enlarged nerves herald leprosy. Tender nerves may be a sign of reaction and warrant immediate action. Inexperienced examiners should learn to palpate at least the ulnar, the radiocutaneous and the great auricular nerves.

When someone has nodules or papules which are skin coloured and firm on palpation, leprosy should be suspected, especially when these are symmetrically distributed on the colder parts of the body, such as ears, nose, cheeks, elbows, buttocks and knees. A skin smear or biopsy should be positive for *M. leprae*. The presence of enlarged nerves may be helpful. Improper closure of an eyelid and dry spots on the skin of palms or soles may also indicate leprosy and warrant further investigation. The same – of course – applies in the case of lagophthalmus, claw hands, drop feet, painless blisters and ulcers, but then severe damage has already occurred.

Classification may be difficult. In short:

1   Paucibacillary features are loss of sensation in a well-defined patch with central healing. The patches are few (less than 3-5) and asymmetrically distributed. Only one, maximum 2 nerves may be enlarged or show signs of neuropathy.
2   Multibacillary features are papules and nodules and/or ill-defined patches with a symmetrical distribution. In particular, small papules may be present along the ears; the earlobes may be swollen and sometimes a lateral madurosis (loss of eyebrows) is present; skin smears are positive. Nerves are symmetrically involved and enlarged (8).

7.5 LABORATORY TESTS

There are no laboratory tests sensitive enough to replace an expert leprologist. Serology, especially against phenolic glycolipid I (PGL-I), can be used for the follow-up of an individual multibacillary patient during treatment, in the same way as the bacterial index (BI) (logarithmic representation of the count of acid-fast bacteria in a for AFB stained skin smear) is used (9). Serology may be positive in contacts and negative in PB patients. PCR and NASBA may detect *M. leprae* DNA and RNA in all untreated MB patients and often detect them in PB patients too, but certainly not always (10).

Skin tests, in particular the well-known lepromin test, may be of assistance in the classification, being positive in tuberculoid and negative in lepromatous patients.

However, it can be positive in leprosy contacts and even in leprosy non-contacts. The same applies for laboratory tests such as the Lymphocyte Transformation Test. Lepromin is obtained from biological material such as human and armadillo; therefore it is difficult to obtain. Its use is sometimes debated, since it may be contaminated with human or armadillo proteins.

Histopathology is an important and sensitive diagnostic tool, but still the experienced physician remains the 'golden standard'.

7.6 DIAGNOSIS OF REACTIONS

The recognition of reactions is of utmost importance since the reactions may lead to permanent nerve damage and functional impairment (11). Two reactions may occur:

The Type-I leprosy reaction also called Reversal Reaction (RR), a typical Gell and Coombs type IV immune reaction, and,

Figure 7.5   Reversal Reaction: swollen erythematous enlarged lesions

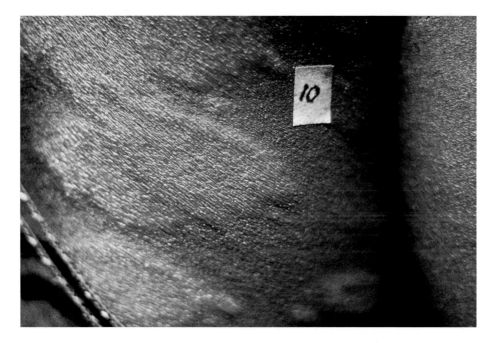

The Type-II leprosy reaction also called Erythema Nodosum Leprosum (ENL), which seemed to be caused by the formation of immune complexes within the tissues (Gell and Coombs type III immune reaction).

A RR can be suspected when a lesion becomes more inflamed, becoming red and swollen, and enlarges (figure 7.5). New patches may appear, especially in MB leprosy. In these patients acroedema may also occur. Nerve lesions may manifest themselves with increasing loss of sensation and strength. Patients may complain of neurological pains. Nerves may enlarge, becoming palpable and tender (11).

ENL is a reaction that occurs mainly in MB patients with an established leprosy infection of longer duration. It may be a generalised reaction accompanied by fever and discomfort. The patient is usually ill and shows painful erythematous or skin coloured papules and nodules, which are tender on palpation (figure 7.6).

Figure 7.6   Erythema Nodosum Leprosum (ENL)

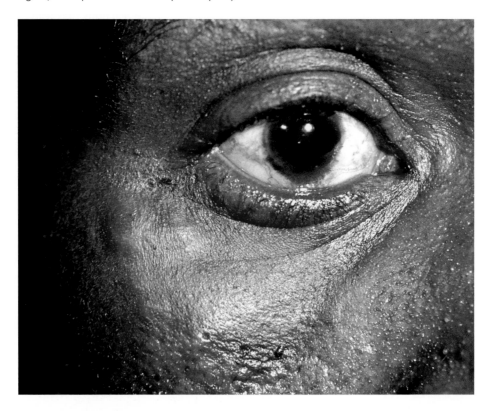

The lesions often are more easily palpated than seen. The lesions are most commonly situated on the extremities and in the face. ENL, being a generalised disease, may also show neuritis, lymphadenitis, arthritis, orchitis, keratitis, iridocyclitis (cave glaucoma), glomerulonephritis and hepatitis. Even peritonitis has been observed. Each of these symptoms may occur separately or in any combination. ENL is an episodic phenomenon. It occurs and abates apparently spontaneously. More than 90%

lasts less than one month. When it becomes chronic the possibility of a simultaneously occurring tuberculosis infection should be considered and excluded (11).

Both reactions may occur before antimycobacterial treatment is instigated, during treatment and even after treatment, when a patient is bacteriologically cured but is still immunologically active. Reactions belong to the natural course of a leprosy infection. However, antimycobacterial treatment may either precipitate a reaction or prevent it, but it is certainly not the cause.

7.7 ANTIMYCOBACTERIAL TREATMENT

Until recently two types of treatment regimes were given: one to PB patients and the other to MB patients. The results of these regimes were excellent; hardly any relapses occurred (7,8).

Paucibacillary leprosy patients received 6 monthly dosages within 9 months, for an adult 600 mg rifampicin once monthly supervised and 100 mg dapsone daily unsupervised. Children received dosage according to weight. For a white adult Caucasian a maximum dose of 50 mg dapsone may be considered since haemolysis among this group occurs regularly and is not only related to G6PD deficiency.

Multibacillary leprosy patients received in addition once monthly 300 mg clofazimine (Lampren®) under supervision and daily 50 mg clofazimine unsupervised. (When 50 mg clofazimine is not available, 100 mg alternate days may be given). Within 36 months 24 dosages should be given.

In 1998 WHO gave new directions. It recommended for Single Lesion Leprosy a single dose treatment consisting of rifampicin 600 mg, ofloxacin 400 mg and minocycline 100 mg (ROM-treatment). For children this should be adjusted to age and weight.

Single Lesion Leprosy is often seen in children. It heals spontaneously in over 80%. It is frequently indeterminate leprosy which, when it does not heal and is left untreated, may go into frank tuberculoid or lepromatous leprosy. Whether this single dose treatment will be effective for the not self-healing Single Lesion Leprosy has not yet been properly established but may be doubted.

For MB patients the WHO recommended shortening the treatment period to only 12 monthly dosages, within 18 months. Strong opposition of the leprologists met this recommendation. They feared relapses, especially in patients with a high number of bacteria, and more severe reactions after the discontinuation of treatment. They advise treating only MB patients with low bacteria count (low BI) with this shortened course of treatment and none of the others (8,9).

7.8 TREATMENT OF REACTIONS

When a Type I leprosy reaction (RR) occurs, prednisolone has to be added to the antimycobacterial treatment, to start with 0.5-1 mg per kg bodyweight in a single morning dose daily. Some may argue that steroids are a dangerous treatment, but they should realise that if left untreated a RR may lead to lifelong disability, which does not occur when properly treated. When the reaction settles, the prednisolone treatment can be slowly tapered off but should, for at least 3-6 months, remain above 0.25 mg/kg. Thereafter it can be tapered off further under careful observation of the nerve function. Voluntary muscle testing (VMT) and graded sensory testing (GST) are extremely useful instruments for this. In patients with a contraindication for the use of steroids cyclosporin may be considered (11,12).

It must be noted that a RR regularly occurs after the discontinuation of the anti-mycobacterial treatment, probably due to the discontinuation of dapsone, which has immunomodulating properties. A reaction occurring after treatment should also be treated with steroids. It is either an autoimmune reaction against antigenic determinants on the patients' own tissue which are identical to those of *M. leprae*, or a reaction against remnant *M. leprae* antigens.

It is advisable to check on parasites (worm) infections before the steroid treatment is started. However, this should not delay the treatment (11,12,13).

An ENL reaction is an episodic phenomenon and should be treated when it occurs. Dr. Souza Araújo in 1929 has noted the natural duration of the reaction: most reactions last only 2 weeks, nearly all end before a month has passed.

A mild reaction, with some discomfort and a few ENL nodules, responds to mild anti-inflammatories and analgesics. It usually will abate spontaneously. However, when it is more severe or involves eyes or nerves, steroids are indicated, since damage may occur that might be irreversible. Mostly a dosage of 1 mg/kg suffices. It can be tapered off in 2-4 weeks time, the natural course of the reaction. In more severe reactions especially in patients with chronic and recurrent reactions the treatment should be started with 2 mg/kg and tapered down quickly in 3-4 weeks. In case the reaction reoccurs, treatment should be restarted at full dose. When it occurs during tapering off one may consider only doubling the dose. A long and continuous maintenance dose of steroids should be prevented (11,12).

When a reaction becomes chronic a careful search for a possible underlying illness should be done. When a cause cannot be found, a long-term course of thalidomide has to be instigated and it is advisable to use clofazimine as well, to start with 300 mg daily which can be tapered of over a period of 3-6 month to 100 mg. Thalidomide may also be used in the treatment of acute ENL reactions. (Starting doses 100-300 mg). But since this, due to its history, is not easily available it should be reserved for the chronic recurrent cases. Recently it was suggested that TNF-α was the crucial molecule in the pathogenesis of ENL. For that reason for a period pentoxifylline was advised for treatment but that showed to be not very active. One of us (Faber) used with success a biological TNF-α inhibitor, infliximab, in a patient with chronic ENL. After more than 1 year no recurrence was seen.

If during a RR or ENL a nerve continues to deteriorate despite adequate treatment where other nerves recover, a nerve release operation should be considered. This should be done under steroid coverage.

7.9 REHABILITATION AND PREVENTION

After nerve damage has occurred and has become irreversible, proper care should be taken. This includes health education and physiotherapy to keep the hands mobile, the eye protected and the foot covered with suitable footwear. Dropfoot surgery, eye and hand surgery can be contemplated. This is often successful in children and young adults when done by experienced surgeons alongside experienced physiotherapists and health educators (11).

REFERENCES

1   Lockwood DN, Suneetha S. Leprosy: too complex a disease for a simple elimination paradigm. *Bull World Health Organ* 2005;83:230-5.
2   Lockwood DN, Reid AJ. The diagnosis of leprosy is delayed in the United Kingdom. *QJM* 2001;94:207-12.
3   Trindade MA, Manini MI, Masetti JH, Leite MA, Takahashi MD, Naafs B. Leprosy and HIV co-infection in five patients. *Lepr Rev* 2005;76:162-6.
4   Naafs B, Silva E, Vilani-Moreno F, Marcos EC, Nogueira ME, Opromolla DVA. Factors influencing the development of leprosy: An overview. (Editorial). *Int J Lepr* 2001;69:26-33.
5   Ridley DS, Jopling WH. Classification of leprosy according to immunity. A five group system. *Int J Lepr* 1966;34:255-70.
6   Leiker DL. Classification of leprosy. *Lepr Rev* 1966;37:7-13.
7   Lockwood DN, Kumar B. Treatment of leprosy. *BMJ* 2004;328(7454):1447-8.
8   Britton WJ, Lockwood DN. Leprosy. *Lancet* 2004;363(9416):1209-19.
9   Chin-A-Lien RAM, Faber WR, v Rens MM, Leiker DL, Naafs B, Klatser PR. Follow-up of multibacillary leprosy patients using a phenolic glycolipid-I-based ELISA. Do increasing ELISA-values after discontinuation of treatment indicate relapse? *Lepr Rev* 1992;63:21-7.
10 Wit MY de, Faber WR, Krieg SR, Douglas JT, Lucas SB, Montreewasuwat N, Pattyn SR, Hussein R, Ponninghaus JM, Hartskeerl RA, Klatser PR. Application of a polymerase chain reaction for the detection of Mycobacterium leprae in skin tissue. *J Clin Microbiol* 1991;29:906-10.
11 Naafs B. Current views on reactions in leprosy. *Indian J Lepr* 2000;72:97-122.
12 Naafs B. Treatment of reactions and Nerve Damage. *Int J Lepr* 1996;64:S21-8.
13 Naafs B. Treatment duration of reversal reaction: A reappraisal. Back to the past. *Lepr Rev* 2003;74:328-36.

8 Leprosy: disability and rehabilitation

J.W. Brandsma

8.1 INTRODUCTION

Leprosy is an infectious disease that may result in transient or chronic disability, mainly due to nerve function impairment. Early diagnosis and treatment of the disease along with early recognition and appropriate treatment of leprosy reactions that involve the nerves can prevent most disabilities. In this chapter the common disabilities will be presented. Prevention of disabilities will be discussed and, when present, how these can be corrected or progression of deformity avoided.

8.2 TERMINOLOGY AND DEFINITIONS

In this chapter disability terminology as defined by the World Health Organization will be used as published in the International Classification of Disability, Functioning and Health (1).

Impairments are problems in body function or structure such as a significant deviation or lack. *Activity limitations* are difficulties an individual may have in executing activities. *Participation restrictions* are problems an individual may experience in involvement in life situations. Impairments are thus changes in body anatomy, physiology or mental function. Activity limitations are difficulties in functioning at the personal level (Activities of Daily Living) and participation restrictions are problems at the societal, socioeconomic level, including attitudes.

Disability is an umbrella term for impairments, activity limitations and participation restrictions.

Rehabilitation is a dynamic multidisciplinary process, that, in partnership with a client, often combines interventions of medical, social, educational and vocational disciplines to maintain, or obtain and secure, a respected and satisfying place in society, for a person who is experiencing certain problems related to a health condition or disorder (disability).

Case study

A leprosy patient has a right clawhand due to irreversible damage of the ulnar nerve.

Impairments: paralysis and loss of sensation of part of the hand supplied by the ulnar nerve. Possible secondary impairments: contractures, an ulcer, shortening of a finger (absorption).

Activity limitations e.g.: inability to eat, and write properly.

Participation restriction e.g.: may not be allowed to eat with others because of the diseases or may not be able to participate in community activities, often even when medically cured.

8.3 IMPAIRMENTS RELATED TO THE DISEASE AND NERVE FUNCTION IMPAIRMENTS

Most of the common impairments in leprosy are due to nerve function impairment (NFI) as a result of leprosy neuropathy which is often part of a reversal reaction or a type II (ENL) reaction (see Chapter 7 on clinical leprosy). A few impairments e.g.

Figure 8.1   Primary and secondary impairments

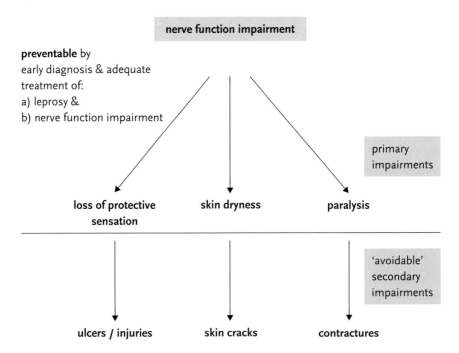

loss of eyebrows and collapse of the nose are seen in lepromatous leprosy but can be prevented by early diagnosis and regular treatment.

Clinically detectable NFI is usually a later occurrence in the course of the disease and can often be prevented by an early diagnosis of the disease or timely detection and treatment of NFI after the start of treatment.

Impairments due to NFI can be classified into primary and secondary. The primary impairments are the direct results of damage to the sensory, motor and autonomic nerve fibres: anaesthesia (loss of feeling), paralysis and loss of sweating. The secondary impairments are the result of 'neglect', e.g. lack of awareness of exercises known to prevent contractures and also the need to change one's lifestyle to prevent injury due to loss of protective sensation (figure 8.1).

Assessment of nerve function

Voluntary muscle testing (VMT) and sensory testing (ST) with nylon monofilaments (or ballpoint pen) should be done at the time of diagnosis and regularly thereafter to establish whether there is some NFI or to find out if NFI may have happened, sometimes unnoticed and insidiously, after diagnosis (figure 8.2).

Figure 8.2   Monofilament testing

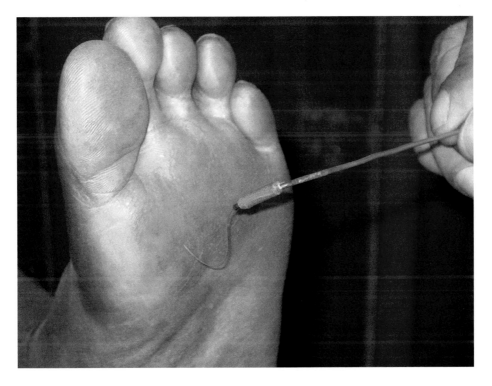

Table 8.1   Nerves at risk in leprosy neuropathy

Nerve	When impaired ...		VMT	ST	Palpation
facial	lagophthalmos		Y	–	–
trigeminal		impaired corneal sensation	–	Y	–
gr. auricular	[1]		–	–	Y
ulnar	claw fingers	impaired sensation	Y	Y	Y
median	loss of thumb opposition	impaired sensation	Y	Y	Y
radial	wrist drop		Y	[2]	Y
comm. peroneal	drop foot	impaired sensation	Y	[3]	Y
post. tibial	claw toes	impaired sensation	[4]	Y	(Y)
sural	[1]		–	[5]	(Y)

VMT: Voluntary Muslce Testing; ST: Sensory Testing: Tested Y = yes; - = negative
1 No significant functional impairment.
2 Radial nerve supplies sensation to the dorsal side of the thumb and the thumb web space. Normally not tested.
3 Common peroneal nerve supplies sensation to the dorsum of the foot. Normally not tested.
4 Posterior tibial nerve supplies all intrinsic muscles of the foot. Normally not tested.
5 Sural nerve is sensory nerve supplying lateral border of the foot. Normally not tested.

VMT and ST are 'proxy' measures which assess to what extent the nerve is functioning. The findings on nerve palpation are of clinical relevance but these findings e.g. enlargement and tenderness are not necessarily related to nerve function.

Nerve function impairment is often reversible and permanent disability can thus be prevented if NFI is detected in time and appropriate treatment started (2,3). The reliability of tests such as those that assess specific muscles and others that assess sensory function at specific sites of nerves that are at risk, have been researched in leprosy and are reported to be very good (4).

Only certain superficial nerves are at risk in leprosy neuropathy. Table 8.1 shows the nerves that are at risk and lists what deformity may result if there is loss of function. It also lists whether the nerve can be assessed for its sensory or motor function and if it is normally palpated for enlargement and tenderness in clinical examination.

Prevention of secondary impairments

One of the more common secondary complications is ulcers, especially plantar ulcers. Hand and eye injuries due to loss of sensation also occur but are less frequent. The etiology and pathomechanics of ulcers and subsequent deformity vary greatly between hands and feet.

Ulcers, and especially chronic longstanding non-healing ulcers, are often a 'stigma' of the disease in leprosy endemic countries (figure 8.3). Ulcers can often be prevented by wearing protective footwear with a soft, microcellular rubber insole. It is important that people who lack protective sensation in their feet, understand that ulcers are not an inevitable consequence of the disease. The health worker should try to find out what may have caused the ulcer. The common answer to the question 'How did you get this ulcer' 'Came by itself' should be taken as a non-answer. It is

Figure 8.3   Foot ulcer (drop foot)

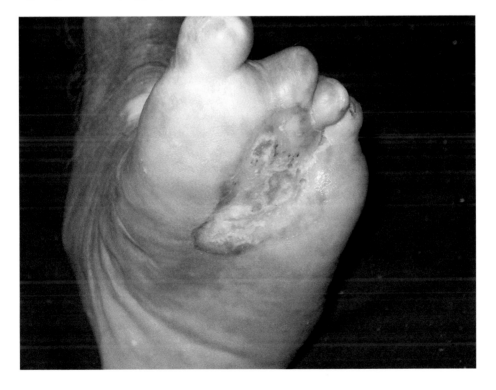

important to find out with the person what was the probable cause. Then action can be taken to prevent recurrence of an ulcer. Has (protective) footwear been used? Has there been a possible burn? Have there been long periods of work in the field without footwear? Has there recently been a very long walk, with/without ill-fitting footwear? Check footwear for irregularities and proper fit. By 'interviewing' the person in this way they should become aware that it is not the fact that they have leprosy that causes ulceration.

Secondary to paralysis and muscle imbalance joint stiffness (contractures) may develop. These are very common in the hand with ulnar paralysis. Paralysis of the posterior tibial nerve and/or common peroneal nerve may result in claw toe deformity. Simple exercises may prevent the occurrence of contracted finger joints and stiff toes (figure 8.4). Mild contractures can also be overcome by exercises.

Eye exercises
Nerve function impairment of the face may lead to the inability to close the eye which is known as lagophthalmos. Often only the zygomatic branch of the facial nerve is affected. Total facial palsy is not as common as lagophthalmos alone. The eye is

Figure 8.4   Hand exercises

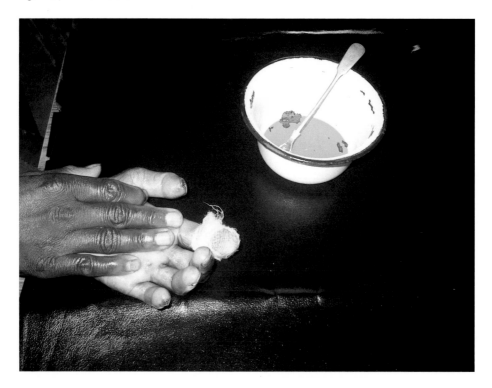

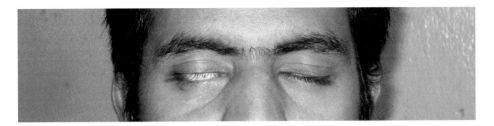

Figure 8.5   Lagophthalmos

especially at risk if there is concomitant impairment of the ophthalmic branch of the trigeminal nerve that supplies sensation to the eyeball. The eye cannot close and the person does not feel when there are offensive particles on the eyeball or when the eye is inflamed (figure 8.5).

Such persons need to be aware that the eye is at risk and they need to inspect their eyes daily. Exercises to strengthen weak muscles may result in complete or near eye closure when there is a minimal lid gap. People with lagophthalmos also need to understand that on attempted eye closure the eyeball will move up under the upper eyelid (Bell's reflex or phenomenon). During the day they will often have to think about closing their eyes regularly, knowing there will not be eye closure but that the eyeball will move under the upper eyelid. This will result in offensive particles being washed from the eyeball and a new tear film will be laid upon the eyeball. This is especially important when it is dusty and windy. (Sun) glasses may be advisable. This will protect the eye from direct sunlight and will prevent offensive particles from entering the eye directly.

Self-care
It is very important that people with insensitive limbs learn that these limbs can serve them a lifetime by taking precautionary measures and making appropriate adjustments in lifestyle. Self-help/support groups of people with insensate feet (diabetes) may be very helpful. People meet regularly to share with one another, show each other their feet (hands), take note of those who may have a problem and discuss how this may have happened and what should be done about it. These self-help groups would often only be feasible and practical when there are a number of people with 'feet-at-risk' living in proximity to one another (5,6).

Surgical correction of primary impairments
The common primary impairments that can be corrected, are the paralytic conditions. All paralytic deformities, resulting from leprosy neuropathy, can be surgically corrected by tendon transfer procedures and other techniques (7) (figure 8.6). These

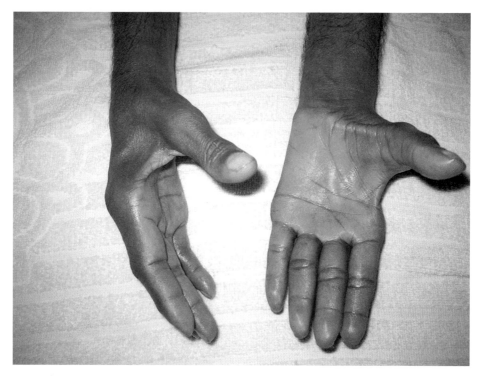

Figure 8.6   Tendon Transfer Surgery Hand

operations should be done by surgeons who have adequate training in leprosy recon-structive surgery. Pre- and postoperative therapy is of utmost importance. Without proper (physio/occupational) therapy postoperatively, maximum potential gains will not be achieved. This applies especially to reconstruction of the paralysed hand. The best results of tendon transfer surgery are obtained in limbs without secondary de-fect e.g. contractures.

Selection of individuals is also important. Persons with paralytic conditions should be motivated to have surgery and should realise that they may not be able to do their regular work for 2-3 months.

Case study
A young women presents with a left hand combined ulnar and median palsy and a right drop foot. There are no secondary impairments of her hand but there is a small ulcer on her foot with some shortening of some of the toes. The left hand is corrected by two tendon transfers in one session.   >>

>> One flexor digitorum superficialis muscle is used to correct the claw finger position. A second tendon is used to correct opposition of the thumb. The hand is in a cast for three weeks. Postoperative therapy is started on cast removal and will take 4 weeks.

Following healing of the small ulcer the drop foot is corrected by transfer of the tibialis posterior tendon. The foot will be immobilised for 4 weeks after which time post-operative therapy will start.

Dealing with secondary impairments and deformities

The common secondary impairments are usually due to the loss of protective sensation in hands and feet. Foot ulcers are the most common secondary impairment. Because of the lack of pain, persons with insensate feet often remain 'mobile'. These ulcers, therefore, often do not heal or do easily recur, especially when there is underlying deformity present. Ulcers can be healed in a variety of ways. Rest is the common denominator (figure 8.7).

Which method is selected depends on such factors as the condition and location of the ulcer, age, profession and motivation.

a   Bed-rest. Not always practised nor practical. The person with an ulcer is generally not sick, does not feel pain and wants to be able to move around, go outside, work on the land, etc.

b   Pair of crutches. These can be given to most people to enable them to remain ambulant.

c   Heelwalking. If an ulcer is located on the forefoot, which is the most common site for an ulcer, especially with only one foot affected, a person can be taught to walk on his/her heel. This presupposes good use of the hands and, naturally, absence of a drop foot deformity.

d   Custom-made footwear or footwear with special inlays. Expertise and workshops are not always available.

Figure 8.7   Rest: the key to healing an ulcer

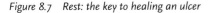
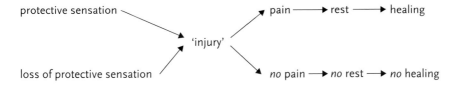

A very effective method for the healing of uncomplicated ulcers is Total Contact Casting (TCC) (7,8). A well-fitting TCC greatly reduces forefoot pressures, allowing the person to remain ambulant. Crutches as with the earlier methods mentioned, are not needed as one cannot be sure that there will not be the occasional 'walk' on the ulcer.

Having given important ways of resting a limb, thereby allowing healing of a plantar ulcer, it is of utmost importance that people with insensate limbs understand why an ulcer has occurred and how reoccurrence of an ulcer may be prevented.

Ulcer surgery

Many foot ulcers may need wound debridement or sequestrectomies to facilitate wound healing. Many wounds can also be surgically closed by skin grafting techniques or transposition flaps. The options are many and the reader is referred to a surgical textbook to get an idea of the full scope of surgical management of plantar ulceration (7).

Foot deformity and/or abnormal foot mechanics may be an important predisposing factor in the (re)occurrence of plantar ulcers. An understanding of normal and deviating foot mechanics is helpful in the management of plantar foot ulcers (9). Special mention is made of the foot with neuropathic bone disintegration also seen in the feet of persons with diabetic neuropathy. With good management, including adequate footwear and lifestyle changes, these feet can also serve a lifetime and amputations can be avoided.

Foot care

In other paragraphs of this chapter important aspects of foot 'disability', both prevention and correction, have been discussed. Feet, in countries where leprosy is endemic, are the most important means of getting from one place to another. Moreover, most people who have (had) leprosy, and, as a result of leprosy neuropathy and who thus may have developed loss of protective sensation of their feet, earn their living standing on their feet, working the land.

It is therefore not surprising that in leprosy hospitals, or wards, in leprosy endemic countries, many of the beds are occupied by leprosy patients with foot problems. Admittedly often they are now the 'elderly' leprosy patients who have had loss of protective sensation for years, many of them with deformed feet, which increases the likelihood of re-ulceration.

Appropriate footwear and change of lifestyle can be very helpful in the (re)occurrence of plantar ulceration but

1   footwear (incl. soft insoles) is not always available, or when available, costly or not always acceptable;

2 achieving a change in lifestyle, 'soak and care for your skin', 'rest an ulcer', 'don't' walk on it', is harder than prescribing a drug.

Self-help or support groups can be very effective in keeping members accountable and reduce the 'burden' of suffering for people with feet-at-risk, and the referral centres for special treatment.

Preventing the first ulcer in newly diagnosed persons with loss of protective sensation of their feet should have first priority. Next priority would be the prevention of a second ulcer in people who have already reported with an ulcer or in whom a first ulcer developed after diagnosis. Most ulcers can be prevented! There is already a great reduction in leprosy patients who at the time of diagnosis present with plantar ulceration or other impairments. Due to better awareness and reduced 'stigma' patients report early for treatment without NFI. All ulcers can be healed, given proper treatment, save the few, often chronic, ulcers in which malignancy may have developed.

Reduction of the number of plantar ulcers and prevention of ulcers remains *the* challenge in many programs that care for and treat people with feet that have loss of protective sensation.

For an up-to-date review of all important aspects regarding etiology, treatment and prevention of plantar ulceration the reader is referred to a recently published textbook (7).

Socioeconomic rehabilitation

Traditionally in many programs, if any socioeconomic assistance was provided, this assistance was usually direct client assistance. A goat or some chickens were given to a client, sometimes a sewing machine or a loan for a business or house. This can still be a very useful thing to do for a well-selected person. Material assistance, however, may help the client to become financially independent, or less financially dependent, but will often not be of any help in '... restoring the client to a respected and satisfying place in society' (see definition of rehabilitation above).

Self-help groups, preferably of a mixed composition of disadvantaged, not necessarily disabled, people may be beneficial in starting small scale income generating, home-based, projects, distributing and controlling loans, being a voice that can be heard in the community etc. Apart from these the self-help groups are helpful in developing self-esteem and self-confidence. It can also just be a platform for disadvantaged people to discuss issues amongst themselves which may help them to solve these issues or direct them to appropriate authorities. In Nepal leprosy-affected persons who are members of a support/self-help group, are generally part of a group of people with different disabilities.

Disability awareness raising at all levels is also a very important strategy in overcoming prejudice, and reducing stigma so that people with disability may become respected persons in society.

In leprosy non-endemic countries the healthcare and social security system will usually be such that expertise is available for custom-made footwear and jobs can be modified or changed.

Disability assessment

To assess to what extent services and interventions are effective in preventing or alleviating disabilities, it is important to assess and evaluate the presence of, and changes in disabilities in individual people affected by leprosy and also in cohorts of persons with the same condition. There are many assessment scales and instruments at the impairment level, all of which are well known and well researched in people affected by leprosy. The more important ones are manual muscle testing and monofilament testing to evaluate nerve function. Other assessment well known in leprosy are the WHO disability grading and vision testing.

These are important assessments, but they do not inform us to what extent people are affected by leprosy experience problems and difficulties in their personal functioning, activities of daily living, and in their social functioning. These are often more of a problem for leprosy patients than the fact that they have physical impairments.

Two scales have been developed in recent years. They have been field-tested and validated in different cultures/countries in, primarily, groups of leprosy patients. The SALSA scale, Screening for Activity Limitation and Safety Awareness, is a scale that will assess to what extent there are difficulties in a number of activities and whether activities are done in a safe manner (10).

The P (Participation) scale is a questionnaire used by an interviewer that will assess if there are problems in the area of socioeconomic functioning and attitudes. These scales have now been validated and are in the process of being introduced in many projects (11,12).

8.4 CONCLUSION

Leprosy disability is primarily related to nerve function impairment. Early diagnosis of the disease and timely recognition and treatment of decreasing nerve function will in most cases prevent irreversible nerve damage. Secondary impairments can be surgically corrected (paralysis) or avoided (ulcers, injuries). Two important scales have been developed that are helpful to evaluate the impact of leprosy related disability on the persons affected by leprosy and to assess the effects of interventions that are directed to remedy the disabilities.

REFERENCES

1   World Health Organization. International Classification of Functioning, Disability and Health (ICF). Geneva: WHO, 2001.

2   Croft RP, Richardus JH, Smith WCS. Field treatment of acute nerve function impairment in leprosy using a standardised corticosteroid regimen- first year's experiences with 100 patients. *Lepr Rev* 1997;68:316-25.

3   Smith WCS, Anderson AM, Withington SG, Brakel van WH, Croft RP, Nicholls RG, Richardes JH. Steroid prophylaxis for prevention of nerve function impairment in leprosy: randomised placebo controlled trial (TRIPOD 1). *Brit Med J* 2004;328:1459-62.

4   Brakel van WH. Peripheral Nerve Function Assessment. In: Schwarz RJ and Brandsma JW (eds.). Surgical Reconstruction and Rehabilitation in Leprosy and other Neuropathies, Nepal Kathmandu: EKTA publishers 2004.

5   Cross H, Newcombe L. An intensive self-care training programme reduces admissions for the treatment of plantar ulcers. *Lepr Rev* 2001;72:276-84.

6   Benbow C, Tamiru T. The experience of self-care groups with people affected by leprosy. *Lepr Rev* 2001;72:311-21.

7   Schwarz RJ, Brandsma JW. Surgical Reconstruction and Rehabilitation in Leprosy and other Neuropathies. EKTA publishers, Kathmandu, Nepal, 2004.

8   Coleman WC, Brand P, Birke JA. The Total Contact Cast. A therapy for plantar ulceration on insensitive feet. *J Am Pod Med Ass* 1984;548-52.

9   Cross H. Biomechanical Assessment of the Foot. In: Surgical Reconstruction and Rehabilitation in Leprosy and other Neuropathies. Schwarz RJ and Brandsma JW eds, EKTA publishers, Kathmandu, Nepal, 2004.

10 The SALSA collaborative study group. The development of a short questionnaire for Screening of Activity Limitations and Safety Awareness (SALSA) in clients affected by leprosy or diabetes. *Disabil rehab,* in press.

11 Anderson AM, Engelbrektsson UB, Khawas I, Kinsella-Bevan S, Grueber M, Mutatkar R, et al. Development of a scale to measure participation. *Int J Lepr* 2002;70 (4):82A.

12 Brakel van WH, Anderson AM, Mutatkar RK, Bakirdtzief Z, Nicholls RG, Raju MS, Das-Pattanayak RK. The Participation Scale – measuring a key concept in international public health. *Disabil Rehab* 2006;28:193-203.

9 Buruli ulcer

F. Portaels and W.M. Meyers

9.1 INTRODUCTION

Buruli ulcer (BU), caused by *Mycobacterium ulcerans*, is an indolent necrotizing disease of the skin, subcutaneous tissue and bone. BU is the third most common mycobacterial disease of humans, after tuberculosis and leprosy, and the least understood of the three diseases.

In 1998 the World Health Organization recognized BU as an emerging health problem, primarily because of its frequent disabling and stigmatizing complications. The disease was named after the geographic area of the first large epidemic investigated in Uganda (in 1961), in a county named 'Buruli' (now called 'Kasongola'), near lake Kyoga.

BU is endemic in Africa, particularly in West African countries. The disease is also endemic outside Africa, but remains uncommon in non-African countries.

In sub-Saharan Africa more than 70% of all patients are children. Individuals 60 years or older are also at increased risk of BU.

The infectious agent, *M. ulcerans*, is an environmental mycobacterium that grows optimally at 30 to 32 °C on mycobacteriologic media such as Löwenstein-Jensen. *M. ulcerans* contains a large plasmid that encodes enzymes which produce a necrotizing toxin, mycolactone, in tissues (1). This toxin diffuses and destroys tissue well beyond the location of the colonies of mycobacteria.

There are genetic and virulence variations in isolates from different geographic origins, with African isolates being much more virulent than those from elsewhere (2).

9.2 EPIDEMIOLOGY

9.2.1 Geographic distribution, incidence and prevalence

BU is focally endemic in rural wetlands of tropical countries of Africa, America, Asia and Australia. A few cases have been reported in non-tropical areas of Australia, Japan and China. Seasonal variations have been reported in Uganda, Papua New Guinea, Cameroon and Australia (3).

Incidence rates vary greatly by continent, country, and in areas within a country. Known incidence rates currently are highest in West Africa, particularly in Benin, Côte d'Ivoire and Ghana. More than 20 000 cases were reported in West Africa during the last decade (4).

In Benin, comparison of detection rates of BU in the Zou region with those of leprosy and tuberculosis in 1999 showed a higher rate of BU (21.5/100 000) than leprosy (13.4/100 000) and tuberculosis (20.0/100 000) (5).

Little is known about the focal epidemiology of BU. Incidence, prevalence, and other data are usually reported at the national or district level. These data show the importance of the disease but do not reveal the wide variations that often exist at the village level within a given district. Prevalence and incidence of BU must therefore be determined at geopolitical divisions below district or national levels (6).

In several countries, over many decades, only a few cases of BU have been reported. In the Americas, the disease seems more common in French Guiana (however, still less than 200 cases over 35 years), than in Surinam, Mexico or Peru, where very few cases have been confirmed. This may be related to gross underreporting, spontaneous healing, environmental and socioeconomic factors, or widespread use of traditional medicine. In Peru some patients showed favorable responses to antituberculous therapy. Although their lesions were extensive, the ulcers were less severe than those often seen in African patients.

The small numbers of BU cases in these countries may be related to a low virulence of the strains of *M. ulcerans* and a more effective immune response of patients. Infrequent contact with contaminated water is clearly not the reason. As in Africa, the populations living in BU endemic areas (e.g. the Amazon basin) have frequent contact with water for domestic use. Similarly, the low incidence of BU in Peru does not seem to be related to the absence of *M. ulcerans* in the environment; IS2404 PCR positivity of the environmental specimens collected in BU endemic foci in Peru (13.8% positivity) and in Benin (10 to 20% positivity) are comparable.

Prevalence of BU is low in Asia and Oceania. Since 1971, more than 400 cases have been detected in Papua New Guinea while in other Asian countries such as Malaysia, China and Japan, only a few cases have been confirmed. In Australia, the disease remains uncommon (4).

9.2.2 Reservoir(s)

The epidemiology of BU is strongly associated with wetlands, especially those with slow-flowing or stagnant water (ponds, backwaters and swamps).

In Benin, we found an inverse relationship between the prevalence of BU and distance from a river. Prevalence in one study increased gradually from 0.6 to 32.6/1000 as the distance from the river decreased from 10 to 1 km. Recently, aquatic insects have been considered potential 'vectors' of *M. ulcerans* (6). These insects can fly many kilometers from their source. This may help explain how patients living some distance from their source of water become infected but not as often as those who live nearer. Considering domestic water sources, only villages near the river used water directly from this river, while other villages employed protected water sources for domestic purposes (boreholes, cisterns, or piped water from artesian wells). These results are similar in Uganda: families who used unprotected sources of water for domestic purposes, had higher prevalence rates of BU than those who used boreholes. Consequently, in addition to the probable influence of distance from the river on disease prevalence through potential carriers such as insects, the use of river water for domestic purposes may play a role in the elevated prevalence rates of the disease in some villages (7).

DNA of *M. ulcerans* has been identified by direct PCR in water and related detritus in Australia, and more recently in aquatic insects, aquatic snails and small fish from endemic areas in Africa (3). Primers targeting the repetitive sequence IS*2404* were used to detect *M. ulcerans* DNA in the environment. This target was considered specific for *M. ulcerans* until recently when several studies reported that mycobacteria other than *M. ulcerans* could harbor the IS*2404* sequence. However, search for environmental *M. ulcerans* DNA in Benin detected variations in positivity rates of aquatic insects (*Hemiptera*) over time, and these changes were reflected in corresponding alterations of frequency of BU patients in the same foci (5). This spatiotemporal relationship between the IS*2404* positivity rates of environmental specimens and the coincident rates of the disease in humans, supports the hypothesis that the IS*2404* positive environmental specimens were positive for *M. ulcerans*.

There is now sufficient evidence from microbiological and epidemiological data (including studies of risk factors) to consider BU as a water-related disease. Aquatic insects, other aquatic invertebrates and fish could be reservoirs or intermediate hosts of *M. ulcerans*.

Despite numerous attempts, *M. ulcerans* had never been cultivated from environmental sources (8) until recently when two pure cultures were obtained form aquatic insects from Benin and from Côte d'Ivoire (6).

9.2.3 Mode(s) of transmission

The exact mode(s) of transmission from the environment and the ultimate natural source(s) of infection remain obscure, and must remain active areas of inquiry. Since the initial discovery of *M. ulcerans* DNA in water bugs in Benin, insects have been suspected as reservoirs for transmission (3,6).

Passage of *M. ulcerans* to mice by the bite of infected water bugs has been reported, suggesting that these insects may play a role in natural transmission (6).

Hemiptera should, however, be considered as 'passive reservoirs' or possible 'vectors'.

Studies on more than 1000 bacteriologically confirmed cases of BU in Benin indicate that trauma is the most frequent means by which *M. ulcerans* is introduced into the human body from the contaminated surface of the skin. Contamination of the skin may result from direct exposure to stagnant water, insect bite, aerosols, or fomites.

Research studies on reservoir(s) and mode(s) of transmission of *M. ulcerans* are urgently needed, especially to develop measures to protect individuals at risk of *M. ulcerans* infection.

9.3 CLINICAL PICTURE

9.3.1 Infection vs disease

Contact with environmental mycobacteria may result in colonization or primary infection of humans or animals. Whether or not this causes clinical disease depends largely on host defenses. It is likely that most individuals exposed to *M. ulcerans* clear the infection and never develop BU disease. Pathogenic mycobacteria including strict pathogens such as *M. tuberculosis* and *M. leprae* or opportunistic pathogens such as environmental mycobacteria, are all capable of establishing persistent infections.

As in tuberculosis, exposure of cutaneous tissues to *M. ulcerans* may lead to early clearance of the infection, development of disease soon after infection (primary BU), or of a subclinical or asymptomatic infection (latent BU) that may subsequently reactivate and produce BU disease.

Mean incubation periods of primary BU are estimated to be 2-3 months. Delayed onset of disease after leaving an endemic area has been seen and probably represents reactivation of latent infection. For example, we have observed individuals who originally resided in a BU endemic area and developed BU at a body site where trauma occurred several years after leaving the endemic area.

Occasionally, the incubation period may be very short (< 15 days). Some patients with such short incubation periods developed the disease after cutaneous trauma without superficial damage to the skin (e.g. bruise or sprain). These cases also suggest reactivation of latent *M. ulcerans* infection by local trauma.

M. ulcerans disease presents in a spectrum of forms related partly to patient delay in admission to hospital. After infection, the disease may become localized by developing a nodule or papule which eventually ulcerates, or may disseminate directly, bypassing the nodular stage. The non-ulcerated form is thus the first stage of the disease in the nodular oedematous, or plaque form. Early stages of the disease are often ignored by the patients, and some may heal spontaneously. After variable periods (a few weeks to several months), these forms ulcerate. Thus, unlike the term 'Buruli ulcer' suggests, the disease does not always present as an ulcer.

9.3.2 **The disease**

Clinically, BU disease may be divided into stages: stages 1 and 2 are active forms, and stage 3 is the healed or scarred lesion. In addition there are mixed forms that appear as combinations of any of the 3 stages at diagnosis.

Non-ulcerated lesions (stage 1)

There are 4 forms characterized as follows:

1   *Nodule*: subcutaneous, firm, palpable, painless or only slightly painful, attached to the skin but not to the deep tissue, up to 3 cm in diameter. The lesion gradually increases in size and is sometimes surrounded by an edematous indurated zone.
2   *Edematous lesion*: a more diffuse, firm, non-pitting swelling, with ill-defined edges, painless or mildly painful and not perceptibly inflamed.
3   *Plaque*: indurated, raised, more or less clearly demarcated, dry, painless and covered with discoloured papery skin.

Figure 9.1   Buruli ulcer puncture wound on abdomen

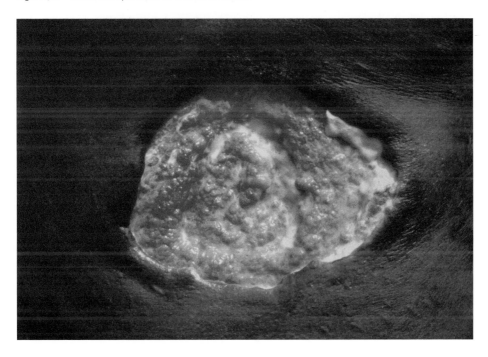

4   *Papule* (most often observed in Australia): raised skin lesion, less than 1 cm in diameter with erythematous surrounding skin.

Ulcerated lesions (stage 2)

More or less extensive single or multiple ulceration, painless or only slightly painful, undermined, with a centre lined with yellowish-white necrotic slough and devitalized edges. The edges are sometimes hyperpigmented. No satellite adenopathies. These lesions are chronic and rarely heal spontaneously. Figure 9.1 shows a typical ulcer with undermined edges.

Figure 9.2   Scarring lesion alongside an ulcerative lesion at the same site (left leg)

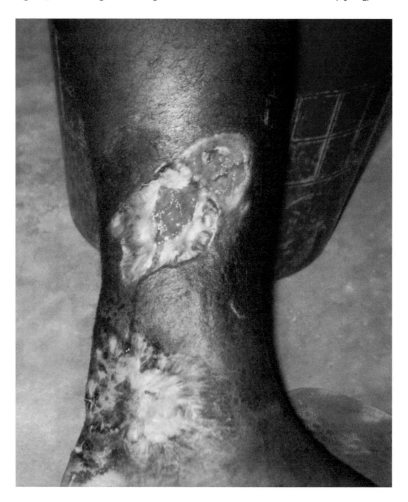

Scar lesions (stage 3)

Atrophic scar, generally following stages 1 or 2. When this develops over a joint, it may lead to severely disabling sequelae. As a result of the adhesion and shrinking of periarticular scars, the range of joint movement is reduced and joints may ankylose and become totally immobile.

Mixed forms

Some patients present mixed forms: the simultaneous presence of different forms in the same patient, at the same or different sites. When the lesions are on different parts of the body they usually represent disseminated forms.

Figure 9.2 shows a mixed form with scarring lesion (inactive) alongside an ulcerative lesion (active) at the same site (left leg).

Disseminated forms

Disseminated forms are characterized by the presence of clinical forms which may or may not be similarly situated at different places on the body. The concept of dissemination denotes spreading of the disease to other parts of the body by contiguous spread or septic metastasis. It is therefore important to examine the patient all over, looking for new or old lesions since the patient may not always be aware of scars of

Figure 9.3   Disseminate form: both legs are affected

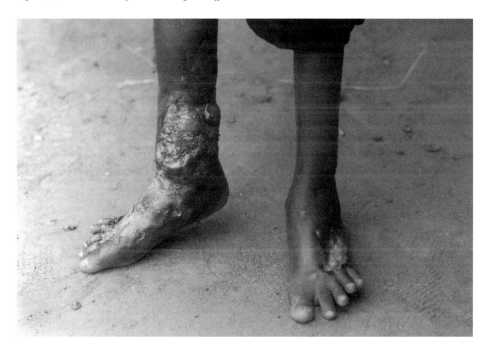

healed infections, for example. Figure 9.3 shows a disseminated lesion: there is an ulcer on the right leg which followed the scarring lesion on the left foot.

Osseous forms
The bacterium infects the bone by 2 different routes:

1   *by contiguity*: *M. ulcerans* reaches the periosteal tissue and bone directly from a BU lesion in the overlying skin and subcutaneous tissue;
2   *by septicemic metastasis*: in this case, infection of soft tissues surrounding the bone is secondary to infection arising within the bone; this occurs at a distance from the initial skin lesion which may already have formed a scar, and of which the patient may be unaware.

Figure 9.4 shows an osteomyelitis of a tibia with eroded bone trabecula and AFB, present in varying numbers in the necrotic bone marrow.

A diagnosis of osteomyelitis should be suspected in the following conditions: presence of edema, slight discomfort early but subsequently painful, with functional disability. Diagnosis is best made by radiological examination.

Figure 9.4   *Osteomyelitis of tibia showing eroded bone trabecula and varying numbers of AFB in the necrotic bone marrow (ZN stain x 100)*

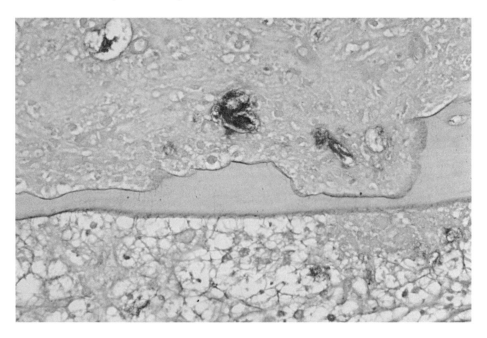

If possible these patients should be referred without delay to the nearest recognized treatment centre for appropriate management. Delay in referral increases the risk for serious consequences such as amputation of limbs.

Frequency of the different clinical forms

The frequency of the different forms varies according to geographic areas, early detection rates and the delay between onset of disease and admission to a BU treatment center. A recent study in a rural hospital of southern Benin showed that the percentages of ulcerated and non-ulcerated forms were each approximately 50% (5). Delayed admission to the hospital results in an increased frequency of ulcerated forms compared to non-ulcerated forms.

9.4 DIAGNOSTIC PROCEDURES

The experienced health worker in endemic areas usually can make an accurate clinical diagnosis.

Clinical criteria for suspecting BU include:

1   presence of a chronically developing lesion (several weeks or months), i.e. a 'wound that will not heal';
2   no fever or regional lymphadenopathy;
3   typical nodular, indurated plaque or edematous lesion;
4   one or more painless chronic ulcers with undermined edges or a depressed scar (there may be pain, fever and even swollen lymph nodes when there is superinfection of the lesion by other bacteria);
5   swelling over a painful joint, suggesting bone involvement;
6   patient age < 15 years;
7   patient living or traveling in an endemic zone.

Microbiologic confirmation of BU is essential for several reasons. Among these reasons are:

1   determination of the true prevalence and incidence of BU in a given area;
2   confirmation of new foci;
3   appropriate management of the disease (by surgery and/or by drug therapy). This is becoming particularly important now that an increasing number of health professionals are using or planning to use antimycobacterial drugs to treat BU.

The clinical diagnosis of BU is usually easy when a child from a known endemic area presents with a typical painless ulcer characterized by undermined edges. Diagnosis should even be easier when health professionals dealing with BU are highly experienced and skilled.

It has now been demonstrated that in regions where health professionals are not highly experienced, few clinically diagnosed or suspected cases are confirmed by laboratory tests. In a study performed in Ghana, where health professionals were trained to recognize and treat early BU lesions, the accuracy of the clinical diagnosis of nodules in these 'experienced' hands, was 48% to 52%.

In another study performed in Côte d'Ivoire, also by 'experienced' health professionals, the accuracy of clinical diagnosis of early lesions was 30%. Among the 70% of misdiagnosed BU, histopathologic analyses performed at the Armed Forces Institute of Pathology, Washington DC, confirmed various types of cutaneous cysts (e.g. epidermoid cysts), Kaposi sarcoma, onchocerciasis, nonspecific chronic inflammation, calcinosis cutis, staphylococcal abscess, phaeohyphomycosis, dermatophytosis, leiomyoma (benign smooth muscle tumor) and even tuberculous lymphadenitis. This list is presented only to indicate that the clinical differential diagnosis of nodular forms of BU can be difficult, even for 'experienced' health professionals. Consequently, the number of declared BU cases may be overestimated, and management of patients with diseases other than BU can be totally inadequate.

Four laboratory tests are currently available to confirm the clinical diagnosis of BU:
1   direct smear examination for acid-fast bacilli (AFB) i.e. Ziehl-Neelsen (ZN) and auramine stain;
2   in vitro culture;
3   IS2404 PCR;
4   histopathological examination.

These tests are described in detail in a freely available WHO manual (9). In endemic areas, the most often available diagnostic technique is the direct smear examination. Culture and histopathology are not widely available in regions were BU is endemic, and PCR can only be performed in well-equipped reference laboratories highly experienced in molecular techniques.

WHO recommends that at least two different laboratory tests be positive to consider a patient as a confirmed BU case.

Two positive tests are preferable to avoid misdiagnosis due to false positive or false negative results and should be required for confirmation of new BU foci, and when health professionals are not highly experienced in the clinical diagnosis of BU. When health professionals are highly experienced, however, one positive test may be sufficient to confirm the diagnosis of BU. Given the heterogeneous distribution of the mycobacteria in the lesions, we also advise that two tissue fragments from excised tissues or two punch biopsy specimens be studied to confirm the clinical diagnosis of BU. As with all laboratory tests, the positivity of the tests depends on the quality of the samples and their prompt delivery to the laboratory.

Laboratory analysis of > 1000 BU proven cases using a strict definition of having at least two different laboratory tests positive, gave a sensitivity of 60 to 80% for ZN staining for AFB, 20 to 80% for culture and > 90% for PCR and histopathology. Indeed, the positivity of the laboratory tests may vary according to the clinical forms. Direct smear examination and culture are less frequently positive for nodules (60% positivity) than for edematous forms (80% positivity). *M. ulcerans* is particularly difficult to cultivate from bone (only 20% positivity).

There is no difference in the positivity of PCR and histopathology results between the different clinical forms (> 90% positivity).

Mycobacteria other than *M. ulcerans* could harbor the IS2404 sequence, but it does not interfere with the diagnosis of BU by PCR as there is no evidence that these *M. ulcerans*-like mycobacteria cause BU in humans.

9.5 **TREATMENT**

Currently, excisional surgery with or without skin grafting remains the recommended therapy of BU. In 2001 WHO published a manual for the surgical management of the different clinical forms of BU (10).

Drug treatment has usually been considered ineffective, although there have been anecdotal accounts of successful antibiotic therapy of early lesions. A number of prospective therapeutic drug trials are presently underway and some are promising.

Provisional guidelines proposed by WHO recommend the use of rifampicin plus streptomycin combined or not with surgery for the treatment of BU (11).

Several centers in Africa have started to treat patients with antibiotics according to WHO guidelines (11) and some studies seem to indicate that following drug therapy for 8 weeks ulcers may heal without surgery. Recurrence rates within the year following the end of treatment were less than 3%. These encouraging results, however, need to be confirmed on a larger number of patients with different clinical forms of BU, and recurrence rates should be evaluated after a follow-up of more than one year.

In a rural hospital of Benin, antimycobacterial therapy was administered as an adjunct to surgery for one week before surgery and continued after surgery for a total of 8 weeks. This study did not show any benefit compared to surgery alone. Antimycobacterial treatment of patients with osteomyelitis did not prevent dissemination to other bones after surgery. Despite some reported encouraging results, additional studies are required to determine the role of antimycobacterial drugs and their optimal use in the management of all clinical forms of BU.

The following aspects of treatment should be further investigated:
1   the duration of antibiotic treatment before and/or after surgery;

2   the possible use of an all-oral regimen;
3   the effect of antimycobacterial therapy without surgery on the regression and
    healing of lesions;
4   the effect of antimycobacterial therapy before surgery on the extent of surgical
    excision (when surgery is required);
5   the effect of antimycobacterial therapy on recurrence rates.

9.6 PREVENTION

In tropical rural settings where BU is endemic and scantily dressed people play and work, avoiding contact with the *M. ulcerans* contaminated environment is virtually impossible. Wearing protective clothing when farming and immediate cleansing of any skin injury may reduce rates of infection, but achieving these measures are seldom feasible.

The use of protected sources of water for domestic purposes reduces exposure to *M. ulcerans* contaminated sources and consequently may reduce prevalence rates of BU (7). Strategies that include drilling wells and supplying pumps, should be developed to provide protected water sources to villages at risk of BU. The problem of reducing risk factors for basic agricultural workers, fishermen and others who must put themselves at risk, remains, however, a serious concern. Appropriate educational programs for behavioral changes, although difficult to implement, should be included in all BU control strategies.

Vaccination programs remain the only viable prevention alternative. Short-term protective effect of BCG has been demonstrated in Uganda, and neonatal vaccination with BCG seemed to reduce the rate of osteomyelitis in BU patients. However, in two recent case-controlled studies performed in Benin, there was no evidence of a protective effect of BCG vaccination against BU (DeBacker et al. and Nackers et al., to be published).

Serious consideration of vaccination rationales should remain a topic of utmost concern in all BU control efforts.

9.7 CONCLUSION

Since BU was declared an emerging disease in 1998, much effort has been invested in research. Some aspects, however, remain unclear and thus require much more investigation, including reservoir(s) and mode(s) of transmission, risk factors, optimal management and preventive tools. BU remains inadequately recognized or understood by health professionals, both within and outside of endemic countries. Thus, research interests and funding are negatively influenced. Moreover, BU is not included in the health statistics of the majority of affected countries. Better strategies for early diagnosis and effective therapy compatible with the socioeconomic structures of BU endemic areas, should be developed. A multidisciplinary approach and productive cooperation between scientists and health professionals remain indispensable for the improvement of BU control worldwide.

Acknowledgement

This work was partly supported by the Damien Foundation (Brussels, Belgium) and by the Directorate-General for Development and Cooperation (Brussels, Belgium).

REFERENCES

1   Stinear TP, Mve-Obiang A, Small PLC, et al. Giant plasmid-encoded polyketide synthases produce the macrolide toxin of *Mycobacterium ulcerans*. *Proc Natl Acad Scie USA* 2004;101:1345-9.

2   Stragier P, Ablordey A, Meyers WM, Portaels F. Genotyping *Mycobacterium ulcerans* and *Mycobacterium marinum* using mycobacterial interspersed repetitive units. *J Bacteriol* 2005;187:1639-47.

3   Portaels F, Chemlal K, Elsen P, et al. *Mycobacterium ulcerans* in wild animals. In: Collins MT, Manning B (eds). Mycobacterial infections in domestic and wild animals. Paris: Office International des Epizooties. Scientific and Technical Review, 2001;20:252-64.

4   World Health Organization. Buruli ulcer disease. *Mycobacterium ulcerans* infection: an overview of reported cases globally. *Wkly Epidemiol Rec* 2004;79:193-200.

5   Debacker M, Aguiar J, Steunou C, et al. Mycobacterium ulcerans Disease (Buruli ulcer) in a Rural Hospital, Southern Benin, 1997-2001. Emerging Infect Dis 2004;10:1391-8.

6   Marsollier L, Robert R, Aubry J, et al. Aquatic insects as a vector for *Mycobacterium ulcerans*. *Appl Environ Microbiol* 2002;68:4623-8.

7   Johnson RC, Sopoh GE, Boko M, et al. Distribution de l'infection à *Mycobacterium ulcerans* (ulcère de Buruli) dans la commune de Lalo au Bénin. *Trop Med Int Health* 2005;10:863-71.

8   Portaels F. Epidemiology of mycobacterial diseases. In: M. Schuster (ed.). Mycobacterial diseases of the skin. Clinics in Dermatology. New York: Elsevier Sciences Inc, 1995;13:207-22.

9   Portaels F, Johnson P, Meyers WM (eds.). Buruli ulcer: Diagnosis of *Mycobacterium ulcerans* disease. Geneva: World Health Organization, 2001.

10 Buntine J, Crofts K (eds.). Buruli ulcer: Management of *Mycobacterium ulcerans* disease. Geneva: World Health Organization, 2001.

11 World Health Organization. Provisional guidance on the role specific antibiotics in the management of *Mycobacterium ulcerans* disease (Buruli ulcer). Geneva: World Health Organization, 2004.

10 Ulcerating pyoderma

J.E. Zeegelaar

10.1 INTRODUCTION

The term pyoderma covers several clinically distinct skin lesions that are mainly due to *Staphylococcus aureus* or β-hemolytic streptococci group A. It is a common cause of (purulent) ulcerative skin lesions in the tropics (1).

In departments for tropical and imported skin diseases, serious (ulcerating) pyodermas, especially of the lower legs, are regularly seen in travellers. As far as we know, the exact incidence of these pyodermas is not known. It is also not known whether the prevalence of bacteria that cause these pyodermas like streptococci and staphylococci, is higher in the tropics or that these bacteria are more virulent. In general, there seems to be no difference in colonization of chronic wounds in the tropics compared to the developed temperate regions of the world. The prevalence of antimicrobial resistance, however, which is high at some locations in the tropics, may complicate treatment. Microcirculatory disturbances leading to subclinical espe-

Figure 10.1   Flowchart: most common causes of ulcerating tropical infection

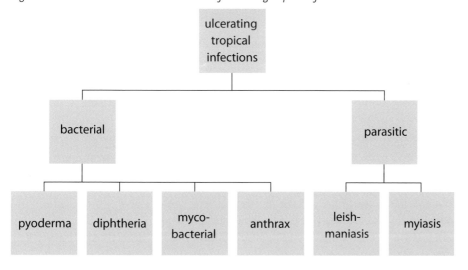

cially at the lower legs has been noticed in travellers. This may delay wound healing in travellers (2).

The most common infectious causes of ulcerations are shown in the flow chart (figure 10.1). In travellers leishmaniasis should always be considered, diphtheria is probably often overlooked (3,4). In this chapter pyoderma and cutaneous diphteria will be discussed.

10.2 EPIDEMIOLOGY

Although ulcerating pyoderma is seen all over the world, it seems to be more prevalent in the tropics. Environmental circumstances such as temperature and humidity may contribute. However, there are only few published studies available on the prevalence or incidence of pyoderma under tropical conditions. A study performed in Blantyre, Malawi, did not reveal a high incidence of ulcerating pyoderma in the in- and out-patient population of the hospital. However, ulcerating pyoderma was the most common cause of these ulcers (5).

β-haemolytic streptococci are carried in the throat by about 10% of the normal population.

β-haemolytic streptococci group A are transmitted mainly through the air by droplets when there is close contact between individuals. Skin lesions and the upper respiratory tract are the primary focal sites of infection. The normal undamaged skin does not provide a favourable habitat. It seems that at least minor trauma is necessary for the development of streptococcal pyoderma. Because under tropical conditions protecting clothing is less used, minor trauma of the skin is more likely to occur, providing an entry for infection.

Colonization of the human skin by *Staphylococcus aureus* is found in 30-50% of healthy adults, with 10-20 % persistently colonized. Carriage sites are the anterior nares, perineum, axillae and toe webs. Infection may be initiated after colonization of skin lesions, especially moist lesions. Whether an infection is contained or spreads depends on several complex factors such as host defence mechanisms and virulence of the *Staphylococcus aureus*. Several toxins and enzymes such as protease, lipase and hyaluronidase contribute to invasion and destruction of tissues. It is not known whether colonization of the skin is higher in the tropics. There has been a worldwide increase of Staphylococcal infections. Systematic surveillance data on prevalence from tropical countries are, however, limited. Some data are available on antimicrobial resistance, which shows methicillin resistant strains as a growing problem. Studies on virulence of these microorganisms have not been published.

Cutaneous diphtheria is still endemic in tropical countries, it is currently rare in the developed world because of the routine practice of active immunization and is mostly travel related. Recent large epidemics in Eastern Europe have again drawn

attention to the disease.With increasing travel to and from endemic countries cutaneous diphtheria may be seen more often in the near future.

10.3 CLINICAL ASPECT

Staphylococcus aureus and group A β-haemolytic streptococcus remain the 2 major
micro-organisms responsible for most ulcerating skin infections. Infection of the
skin with *Staphylococcus aureus* or group A β-haemolytic streptococcus may show different clinical pictures from folliculitis to true skin ulcers (figures 10.2 and 10.3).

Ecthyma is known as a clinical entity and is characterized by a deep pyogenic ulcerating infection. It usually starts as a vesicle or vesiculopustule on an erythematous

Figure 10.2   Healing ulcerating pyoderma with satellite lesions

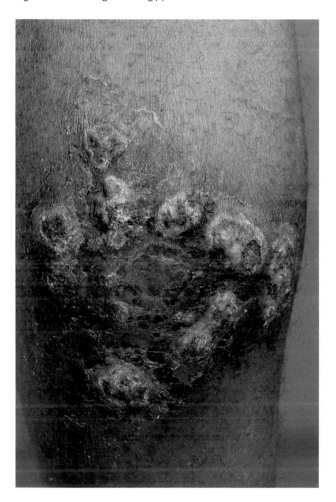

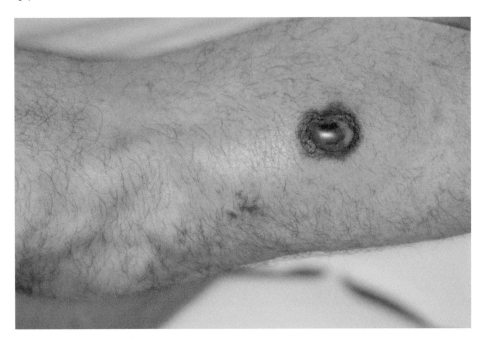

Figure 10.3   Bullous pyoderma with surrounding erythema at the lower leg in a traveller

Figure 10.4   Multiple punched out lesions on the dorsal foot in a traveller

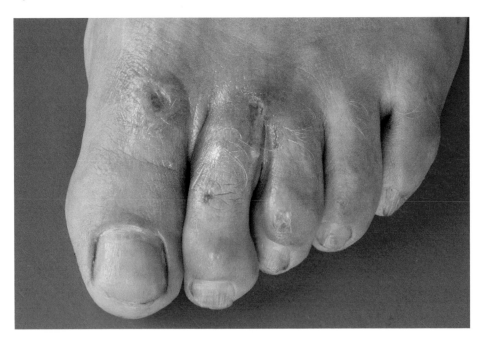

base, which consequently ulcerates. The ulcer is covered with a dark-brown, bloody crust. After removing the crust a tender punched-out ulcer remains. It is usually found on the dorsal feet, shins, thighs and less often on the upper part of the body (figure 10.4). There are usually few lesions and new lesions may develop without adequate treatment. In many ulcers both β-haemolytic streptococci as well as *Staphylococcus aureus* can be found. However, β-haemolytic streptococci are thought to be the primary pathogen.

Pyoderma in travellers is most commonly seen as a secondary infection in skin lesions caused by environmental insults to the skin, such as insect bites, abrasions, and atopic dermatitis.

Corynebacterium diphtheriae is found secondary in a pre-existing ulcer as echtyma or as superinfection of eczema (figure 10.5).

In immunized persons systemic toxic complications such as myocarditis and neuritis are rare. Because cutaneous diphtheria is uncommon in non-endemic countries and clinically not very specific, the diagnosis is often missed or made in a late stage. The most typical manifestation is characterized by a chronic, non-healing ulcer(s) with a punched out appearance, slightly undermined and covered by a grey adherent membrane. In the first 2 weeks it is painful, later the lesion becomes painless and after (spontaneous) removal of the adhering crust, the hemorrhagic base appears.

10.4 DIAGNOSIS

The diagnosis of pyoderma is often made on the basis of a clinical picture of persistent painful ulceration especially on the lower legs. If facilities are available one should perform a bacterial culture. Ideally, tissue obtained by biopsy or needle aspiration should be cultured. In daily practice this is often not routinely performed because it is more time consuming and inconvenient to the patient. However, adequate culture results have been found using swabs. The ulcerated lesion should be cleaned thoroughly with saline solution after which specimens from the wound surface and, if possible, from under the margins of the wounds are collected. Preferably susceptibility tests in vitro should be performed. Methicillin resistant *Staphylococcus aureus* and tetracycline resistant streptococci and staphylococci are frequently found in many parts of the tropical world.

Because ulceration caused by *Corynebacterium diphtheriae* is clinically not specific, a high rate of suspicion is necessary. The definitive diagnosis is made by isolating and identifying the organism from the ulcer and demonstrating its toxigenicity. As routine culture procedures will not isolate *Corynebacterium diphtheriae* the physician must inform the laboratory of the suspicion in advance (6).

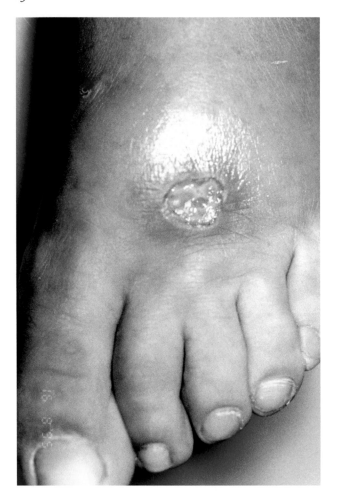

Figure 10.5   Punched out ulcer. Culture revealed β-haemolytic streptococci and C diphtheriae.

10.5 TREATMENT

Treatment of ulcerative pyoderma will be based initially on clinical judgement. Gram-stained smears of exudate may be helpful in order to start empirical antimicrobial treatment. However, preferably, antibiotic treatment should be based on culture results. If culture is not known and the clinical picture demands antibiotic treatment one may start, in cases of community acquired ulcerative pyoderma, with flucloxacillin orally for at least 10 days as drug of first choice. Flucloxacillin is a semisynthetic penicillin. It has a low acute and chronic toxicity, and an a high enteric absorption. The antibacterial activity of flucloxacillin is evident in gram-positive bacteria and above all on penicillinases producing staphylococci. With the global spread of macrolide-resistant *Staphylococcus aureus* and β-haemolytic streptococci, macrolide antibiotics should be prescribed with caution (7). Clindamycin is recommended in penicillin allergic patients. As an alternative vancomycin may be used. However the first vancomycin resistant *Staphylococcus aureus* (VRSA) has been reported.

Besides antimicrobial treatment, local treatment is important and often neglected. It is generally accepted that ulcers heal more rapidly under occlusive (moist) dressings. There are no documented studies in which the effect of these occlusive dressing on healing of ulcerative pyoderma is shown. However, occlusive dressings were shown to be safe in chronic ulcers with an even lower infection rate in occluded wounds compared to ulcers treated with conventional dressings.

Special attention should be given to ulceration of the lower legs in which (sub) clinical edema is often present. This edema may delay or even complicate healing. Edema can be eliminated by adequate compression therapy with elastic or non-elastic bandages.

When there is suspicion of cutaneous diphtheria, treatment should be started as soon as possible. Neutralizing antitoxin, is probably of no value in cutaneous disease. Penicillin and erythromycin are considered drugs of first choice for eradicating *Corynebacterium diphtheriae*.

REFERENCES

1   Mahe A. Bacterial skin infections in a tropical environment. *Curr Opin Infect Dis* 2001;14:123-6.

2   Zeegelaar JE, de Feijter A, de Vries HJ, Lai A Fat RT, Neumann MA, Faber WR. Microcirculatory changes in travelers to a tropical country. *Int J Dermatol* 2002;41:93-5.

3   Zeegelaar JE, Steketee WH, van Thiel PP, Wetsteijn JP, Kager PA., Faber WR. Changing pattern of imported cutaneous leishmaniasis in the Netherlands. *Clin Exp Dermatol* 2005;30:1-5.

4   Black JA. Tropical ulcers and diphtheria. *J R Soc Med* 1998;91:60.

5   Zeegelaar JE, Stroïnk AC, Steketee WH, Faber WR, van der Wal AC, Komolafe IOO, Dzamalala C, Chibwana C, Wendte JF, Zijlstra EE. Etiology and incidence of chronic ulcers in Blantyre, Malawi. *Int J Dermatol* 2006 In press. Digital Object Identifier 10.1111/j. 1365-4632.2006.02858x.

6   Galazka AM, Robertson SE, Oblapenko GP. Resurgence of diphtheria. *Eur J Epidemiol* 1995;11:95-105.

7   Rotta J, Tikhomirov E. Streptococcal diseases worldwide: present status and prospects. *Bull World Health Organ* 1987;65:769-77.

11 Fever and rash

H.G. Schipper and P.A. Kager

11.1 DENGUE

11.1.1 Introduction

Dengue is one of the most important mosquito borne virus infections in the world in terms of morbidity and mortality. Man is infected by the bite of mosquitoes of the *Aedes* genus. Following infection a spectrum of illnesses may occur ranging from unperceivable infection to a severe and fatal disease. Vector control is the most important prevention. Vaccines are not available. Treatment is symptomatic. There is no specific therapeutic agent.

11.1.2 Epidemiology: geographic distribution, mode of infection

The geographic distribution of dengue is primarily determined by the presence of an appropriate vector. Transmission of dengue virus to humans is impossible when the climate in an area is inappropriate for the vector. The dengue viruses are transmitted to man by mosquitoes, primarily *Aedes aegypti* and to a lesser extend by *Aedes albopictus* and *Aedes polynesiensis,* which need a (sub) tropical climate to live. The changing global climate is a potential risk for transmission of dengue in areas which do not harbour these mosquitoes yet, such as the Mediterranean area.

In rare cases, man may also be infected with dengue virus without mosquito bites. Nosocomial transmission of dengue virus was reported following needle stick injuries, bone marrow transplantation, blood transfusion and mucocutaneous contamination. Intrapartum and vertical transmission are possible.

Dengue is endemic in South East Asia, (e.g. Philippines, Indonesia, Thailand, Vietnam, Malaysia), South Asia (Sri Lanka, India), the Far East (China, Fiji, Australia) and the Americas (Cuba, Venezuela and other Latin American countries). Interestingly, some regions are free of disease despite hyper endemic dengue virus transmission. Haiti and Africa are such regions. These observations suggest the presence of a dengue resistance gene in black populations. It is currently estimated that over three billion individuals live in areas at risk for dengue and that each year hundred million cases of dengue fever (DF), half a million cases of dengue hemorrhagic fever (DHF) and thousands of deaths due to DHF occur worldwide. Ninety percent of DHF patients are children less than 15 years of age. Case fatality rate of DHF in Asia is 0.5% to 3.5%.

An increasing number of travellers visiting endemic countries are potentially at risk for being infected with dengue. The risk seems to be low. Only a few studies report on the incidence of dengue infections in travellers to endemic areas; the sero-conversion rates range from 0.3% to 6.7%. Clinical symptoms were reported by less than half of infected cases.

Dengue viruses are members of the *flaviviridae* family, genus flavivirus, and carry a single stranded RNA genome. Four different serotypes were identified: DENV-1, DENV-2, DENV-3, and DENV-4. The DENV-1, DENV-2 and DENV-3 serotypes may cause primary and secondary infections. The DENV-4 serotype is only involved in secondary dengue infections. The serotypes causing epidemic outbreaks in the past are changing. The predominant serotype of major epidemics in the 1980s was DENV-2. In recent years a new subtype of the DENV-3 virus, which originated from India, spread to other continents. This new serotype probably caused a pandemic in a population which was non-immune to this new subtype. In Southeast Asia DENV-1 and DENV-2 were the prevalent serotypes until the late 1980s. DENV-3 serotype was the

Figure 11.1   Dengue hemorrhagic fever in a patient who acquired a secondary dengue infection in Manila/Philippines

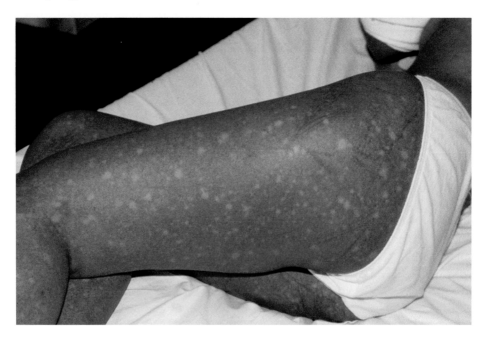

predominant serotype in the recent outbreaks. The changing serotypes which caused epidemic outbreaks were also observed in the Americas. In the late 1970s serotype DEN-1 caused an epidemic in Cuba. The DHF epidemic of 1981 was caused by DEN-2a, mostly due to secondary infections. The current epidemiological trend is similar to that seen in Asia, with DHF epidemics occurring every 3-4 years (1,2,3).

11.1.3 Clinical picture

The incubation period is 3-8 days. Most of the dengue infections are clinically unapparent and indistinguishable from other viral infections. This so-called 'undifferentiated fever' often occurs in infants and young children. The majority of symptomatic cases experiences uncomplicated DF. The most severe cases of DF are usually seen in older children and are characterized by a syndrome with high fever that lasts 2-7 days. Fever may be biphasic or 'saddle back'-like by normalising in the middle of the febrile period. Accompanying symptoms are severe retro-orbital headache, arthralgia, myalgia, anorexia, abdominal discomfort and a rash. Rash may be macular, maculopapular or become diffusely erythematous, sparing small areas of normal skin (figure 11.1).

Severe hemorrhagic manifestations are uncommon but petechiae, purpura, epistaxis, skin bleeding and gastrointestinal bleeding may occur. DF is usually associated with mild to moderate elevations of aminotransferases (about 60% of patients); acute hepatitis may occur in a minority of patients (4%). Levels of aspartate aminotransferase tend to be higher than alanine aminotransferase. Recovery is uneventful and generally occurs after 7-10 days of defervescence. Fatigue may be pronounced for months after resolution of fever.

Dengue hemorrhagic fever (DHF) represents the most severe clinical manifestation of dengue infection and occurs in 2-4% of infected individuals. DHF is usually observed following secondary dengue infections. In Asia, DHF mainly affects children. In the Americas all age groups are affected but the majority of fatalities occur in children. DHF is defined as an acute febrile illness with hemorrhagic manifestations, low platelet count (< 100 x 109/l), evidence of plasma leakage (ascites, pleural effusion, low level of serum albumen) and haemoconcentration (rise of haematocrit by more than 20%). In severe situations, when shock occurs, the disease is called dengue shock syndrome. Convalescence of DHF is usually uneventful. A confluent petechial rash with erythema and islands of pallor (figure 11.1) is characteristic. During recovery, many patients complain of severe itching, especially on the palms and soles, and desquamation (4).

11.1.4 Pathogenesis

An association of increased risk for DHF with a secondary DENV infection was suggested first in seroepidemiological studies in Thailand during the 1960s. To date, this observation is at least partially explained by a complicated mechanism which is unique for dengue virus infections, the so-called antibody dependent enhancement.

Monocytes and macrophages are the primary target for the dengue virus. A primary infection induces antibodies directed to the serotype which causes the primary infection. These antibodies result in a life long immunity to the specific primary serotype and a short lasting cross-immunity to the other serotypes. The dengue virus causing secondary disease is always of a different serotype than the virus that caused the primary infection. During the secondary infection pre-existing T-memory cells and plasma cells are more rapidly activated than naïve B-cells. The levels of pre-existing antibodies are therefore higher than those of the new serotype. The pre-existing IgG antibodies form complexes with the new virus by binding at non-neutralising epitopes. Monocytes, macrophages and other cells are more readily infected by these IgG virion complexes than by 'naked' virions. This phenomenon is called antibody dependent enhancement of infection. Antibody dependent enhancement of infection also explains why infants under one year of age may experience severe infections due to enhancement by the maternally acquired dengue antibodies. This may not be the only mechanism which induces DHF in patients. DHF may also occur in older children and adults with primary infection. Immune complex formation, complement activation, cross reactivity of antibodies against plasminogen, cytokine production and cytolysis by activated T-lymphocytes are additional potential contributors of the disease. Racial differences in susceptibility and possible HLA associations suggest that human genetic factors play a role in pathofysiology. This might explain the absence or rare occurrence of DHF in Haiti and Africa (5).

11.1.5 Diagnosis

Geographical exposition, clinical history and physical examination are the keystones of diagnosis of dengue virus infection. Leucopenia and thrombocytopenia are supportive and serology confirms the diagnosis. Usually, dengue specific IgM and IgG ELISA are used for serological diagnosis. In the first few days of infection ELISA may be negative but most patients have measurable IgM antibodies by the fifth day of infection. IgM antibodies become undetectable at 30-60 days after the onset of illness. IgG antibodies increase shortly after the initial rise of IgM antibodies and remain detectable for life. In secondary infections IgG antibodies are present from the very beginning of onset of disease and rapidly increase. IgM antibodies are generally lower than in primary infections.

Reverse transcriptase polymerase chain reaction (RT-PCR) is a promising new diagnostic tool which also can be used to quantify viral load. Dengue virus culture is not routinely done in diagnostic laboratories.

Abdominal sonography can be used as a first line imaging modality in patients with suspected DF to detect early signs suggestive of the disease. Typical sonographic features of DF include thickened gallbladder wall, ascites, splenomegaly and pleural effusion (4).

11.1.6 Treatment

There is no specific therapeutic agent for dengue viral infections. In mild infections oral hydration and antipyretics can be used such as paracetamol but not aspirin or other non-steroidal inflammatory drugs. Treatment of DHF is also symptomatic and supportive. In severe cases appropriate fluid management to correct hypovolemia is the mainstay of treatment. In patients with dengue shock syndrome, treatment with vasoactive drugs and transfusion of blood, platelets or plasma is frequently necessary (3).

11.1.7 Prevention and control

There is no effective vaccine against dengue yet, but development of a vaccine is in progress. Ideally an optimal vaccine should prevent both DF and DHF. The vaccine should also induce antibodies and T-lymphocytes against all four serotypes to prevent the occurrence of antibody dependent enhancement, if one of the serotypes would not be included in the vaccine.

To date, prevention of mosquito bites and vector control are the only options available. For personal protection against mosquito bites, protective clothing is important but not always practical in tropical climates. Other options are the use of repellents and insecticides. Impregnated bed nets are of little use because *Aedes aegypti* is a day biting mosquito.

Vector control is the main focus of preventing dengue viral infections. *Aedes aegypti* typically rests indoors, mainly in living rooms and bedrooms, and is thereby largely protected from insecticides sprayed outdoors. *Aedes aegypti* easily breeds in all kind of water collections: water containers, polluted water, and small water collections in flower vases, water jars, coconut shells or rubber tyres. Appropriate drinking water and waste water management is therefore crucial in eradication programs. Covering the water jars around the homesteads already is an important measure.

Vector control programs demonstrated their efficacy in Japan and Cuba. These countries became free of dengue. Ongoing vector control programs are vital to control the disease. In the Americas it was demonstrated what occurs when resources for eradication programmes are reduced. These areas became reinfested with *Aedes* mosquitoes and re-emergence of dengue was inevitable (1,3,4).

11.2 RICKETTSIOSES

11.2.1 Introduction

In the past decades rickettsioses have increasingly been diagnosed in travellers to endemic areas. Ecotourism, backpacking, tracking, safari and game hunting and other adventurous activities appear to be risk factors for infection with *Rickettsiae*. Man is infected by arthropods like ticks, mites, flea and lice. *Rickettsiae* are obligate intracellular gram-negative bacteria that invade endothelial cells and cause vasculitis. Rickettsioses are acute febrile illnesses accompanied by headache, myalgia and often a rash. The clinical course is usually benign. Severe complications are rare. The travel behaviour of the tourist and the popularity of the destination largely determine which type of rickettsiosis is acquired, the vast majority being murine typhus (*Rickettsia typhi*), Mediterranean spotted fever (*Rickettsia conorii*), African tick bite fever (*Rickettsia africae*) and scrub typhus (*Orientia tsutsugamushi*). For diagnosis serological tests are widely available. Polymerase Chain Reaction (PCR) can be used additionally. Culture is done only in specified laboratories. Doxycycline is the drug of first choice. Macrolides such as clarithromycine are effective alternatives. Fluoroquinolones are effective in vitro but may fail clinically (6).

11.2.2 Clinical picture, epidemiology

Rickettsioses are divided into three biogroups: typhus group, spotted fever group and scrub typhus (table 11.1).

Table 11.1   Classification into biogroups and diseases of most frequently observed rickettsioses in travellers

Biogroup, Disease	Species	Vector	Geography	Travellers
Typhus				
epidemic typhus	Rickettsia prowazekii	body lice	Central and East Africa, South America	very rare
murine typhus	Rickettsia typhi	rat fleas	tropical and subtropical areas worldwide	occasional
Spotted fever				
Rocky Mountain spotted fever	Rickettsia rickettsii	Dermacentor and Amblyomma ticks	North, Central and South America	very rare
Mediterranean spotted fever	Rickettsia conorii	Rhipicephalus and Haemaphysalis ticks	Mediterranean and Caspian littorals, Middle East, Indian subcontinent, Africa	occasional
African tick bite fever	Rickettsia africae	Amblyomma ticks	rural Sub-Saharan Africa	common
Scrub typhus				
scrub typhus	Orientia tsutsugamushi	chigger mites	Southeast Asia, Western Oceania	occasional

Epidemic typhus

Epidemic typhus, the prototype of rickettsiosis in the typhus biogroup, is caused by *Rickettsia prowazekii* and is rarely diagnosed in travellers. In Dutch it is called 'vlekty-fus'. The disease is transmitted to humans by body lice. For transmission close body contact is necessary. It is a disease of war and concentration camps or refugee camps and of prisons. It is now found in the highlands in East Africa (Ethiopia, Rwanda, Burundi) and could occur elsewhere.

In rare cases, contact with squirrels was reported as the risk factor. Clinical symptoms are fever, constitutional symptoms, maculopapular and petechial rash and in severe cases CNS involvement. Fatality rate may be as high as 40%.

Murine typhus

Murine typhus is the second disease in the typhus group and is caused by *Rickettsia typhi*. Man is infected by rat flea bites. Contact with rats, visits to port cities and beach resorts are possible risk behavior. It occurs in tropical and subtropical areas: Asia (Nepal, India, Thailand, Indonesia, Vietnam, China), Africa (Morocco, Gabon, Botswana, Guinea Bissau) and in Europe (Cyprus, Greece, Spain). The clinical presentation is notoriously non-specific with fever, constitutional symptoms and in about 50% of patients, a poorly visible maculopapular rash. Many patient problems remain undiagnosed or are labeled as fever of unknown origin. The clinical cause is benign. Meningitis, deafness and DVT may occur. Fatality rate is 4%. An inoculation eschar is usually absent.

Mediterranean spotted fever

The most frequently diagnosed diseases of the spotted fever group are Mediterranean spotted fever, African tick bite fever and rarely Rocky Mountain spotted fever. Mediterranean spotted fever is caused by *Rickettsia conorii* and transmitted to man by dog ticks, *Rhipicephalus* and *Haemaphysalis* ticks. Typical risk behavior is contact with dogs in Mediterranean and Caspian littorals. Typical clinical symptoms include fever, constitutional symptoms, a generalized maculopapular rash and an inoculation eschar at the site of the tick bite. In severe diseases CNS involvement may occur and multiple organ failure. Fatality rate is 2%.

African tick bite fever

African tick bite fever is caused by *Rickettsia africae* and transmitted to man by very aggressive cattle ticks, *Amblyomma* ticks. Large parts of rural Sub-Saharan Africa are infected with the ticks. Risk behavior is safari, ecotourism, tracking, adventure race and military activities. Clinical presentation includes fever, constitutional symptoms, one or several inoculation eschars with regional lymphadenitis and a typical vesic-

A B

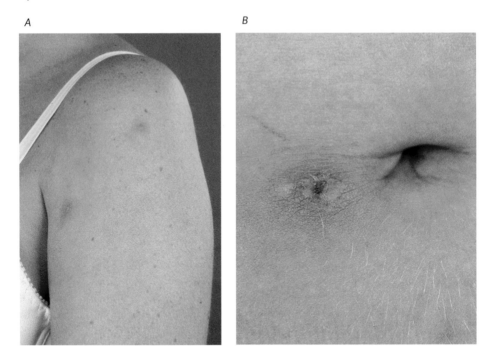

Figure 11.2   A, B African tick bite fever in a female traveller returning from the Kruger Park, South Africa. Typical vesicular rash and an inoculation eschar near the umbilicus.

ular cutaneous rash (figure 11.2A, B) and mouth blisters. African tick bite fever is usually a self-limited mild disease.

Rocky Mountain spotted fever

Rocky Mountain spotted fever is very rarely diagnosed in travellers. Inhabitants of the Southeastern and Midwestern United States and of parts of South America who frequent tick-invested habitats, such as wooded and grassy areas, are at risk for this potentially severe disease. Man is infected by dog tick bites, *Dermacentor* and *Amblyomma* ticks. Characteristic clinical symptoms are fever, headache, and myalgia. An erythematous rash usually starts on ankles and wrists, spreads all over the body and may become hemorrhagic in severe cases (figure 11.3). CNS involvement may occur and multiple organ failure resulting in the death of the patient. An inoculation eschar is usually absent.

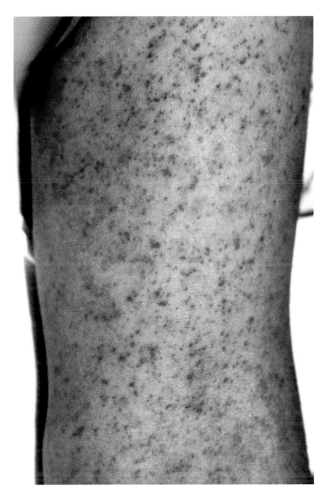

Figure 11.3   Rocky Mountain spotted fever with a maculopapular haemorrhagic rash in a male patient from the South-eastern USA

Scrub typhus

Scrub typhus is endemic in rural South and Southeastern Asia and the Western Pacific. People engaged in logging, working in rice fields and military personnel (World War II; Vietnam War) are at risk. The disease is caused by *Orientia tsutsugamushi*. Man is infected by the bite of larval trombiculid mites (chiggers) that typically bite humans on the lower extremities or in the genital region. Most patients present with fever and generalized lymphadenitis. About half of them have an inoculation eschar. The clinical cause is usually mild, but severe complications may occur such as meningoencephalitis, pneumonitis, renal failure and disseminated intravascular coagulation. Fatality rates range between 1% and 35%. Most travellers become infected in Thailand and less frequently in India, Vietnam, Malaysia and the Philippines (6,7).

11.2.3 Diagnosis
Serology is the diagnostic procedure of choice in rickettsiosis. Blood should be collected early in the cause of the disease with a convalescent phase sample obtained two weeks later. A third sample collected 4-6 weeks after onset of symptoms is helpful if the rise of antibody titers is low (6).

11.2.4 Treatment
Standard treatment of rickettsiosis consists of doxycycline 200 mg daily for 3 to 14 days depending on the severity of the clinical course. Newer macrolides such as clarithromycine 7.5 mg/kg bodyweight twice daily for 7 days are good alternatives. Fluoroquinolones exhibit a good in vitro activity but clinical failure has been suggested in epidemic typhus and murine typhus (8).

11.2.5 Prevention
The best preventive measure is to avoid risk areas and risk behavior or at least to wear protective clothing impregnated with permethrin. Topical repellents have only a short-lasting effect. Weekly dose of doxycycline 200 mg was effective in preventing scrub typhus. Whether chemoprophylaxis is effective in the prevention of other rickettsioses is uncertain (9). Vaccines are not yet available.

11.3 MIGRATORY SWELLINGS

11.3.1 Introduction
With modern-day travel and immigration cases of migratory swellings due to infection with *Gnathostoma* species or *Loa loa* are being diagnosed with increased frequency. The characteristic triad of these infections consists of intermittent migratory swellings, a history of travel to an endemic area and eosinophilia. The geographical history is of crucial importance for the differential diagnosis. Gnathostomiasis is endemic to Southeast Asia and Latin America. Infection with the larvae of *Loa loa* can only be acquired in a limited area in Western and Central Africa.

11.3.2 Gnathostomiasis

Epidemiology, mode of infection
Human gnathostomiasis is caused by *Gnathostoma* species mostly by *G. spinigerum*, less frequently by *G. doloresi, G. hispidum* and *G. nipponicum*. This disease is endemic to a large area in Southeast Asia: India, Thailand, Laos, Cambodia, Myanmar,

Vietnam, Malaysia, Japan, China, the Philippines, Sri Lanka, Indonesia and Australia but also to Latin America, particularly Mexico and Ecuador.

Dogs, cats and cat-likes are the definite hosts that harbour the adult *Gnathostoma* worms in the walls of their stomach. Eggs of these worms develop into first-stage larvae in fresh water and are eaten by copepods (*Cyclops*), the first intermediate host, in the gut of which third-stage larvae develop. Fish, birds and mammals serve as the second-intermediate host when eating infected copepods. Life cycle is closed when definite hosts become infected by eating copepods or second intermediate hosts.

Man is infected by consumption of copepods, undercooked or raw fish, poultry or pork harbouring these infectious larvae (10). In Mexico, gnathostomiasis is strongly connected to a famous traditional dish called 'ceviche', raw fish marinated in lemon juice (11).

Clinical picture

Man is a dead-end-host in whom these third stage larvae do not develop into adult worms. These larvae migrate through the skin and subcutaneous tissues, mimicking creeping eruption or causing migratory swellings often accompanied by fever, localized pain, pruritis, and erythema. In travellers, the time delay from the date of return to their home country to the onset of cutaneous manifestations varied from 10 days to 150 days. The larvae may also migrate to deeper tissues throughout internal viscera causing substantial pain and a broad range of symptoms, depending of the organ involved. Eosinophilia is a marked phenomenon (12).

Diagnosis, treatment, prevention

Serology (ELISA for IgE antibodies) is helpful as a diagnostic test as the definitive diagnosis of identification of the parasite is often not possible. Mebendazole, albendazole, ivermectin and praziquantel are used for treatment but their effectivity is not assured. Relapses may occur 2-24 months after treatment. Drug treatment may cause outward migration of the worm in 5-6% of patients allowing surgical removal, the treatment of choice. Currently, the recommended treatment for gnathostomiasis is albendazole at a dose of 400-800 mg/d for 21 days. The efficacy rate of this treatment was 94%. Prevention is the best therapy for gnathostomiasis. Education of indigenous people and travellers about safe cooking and eating practices is most effective (13).

11.3.3 Loiasis

Epidemiology, mode of infection

Infection with the larvae of *Loa loa* can only be acquired in a limited area in Western and Central Africa where an appropriate vector is present, particularly in the rain forest and swamp forest in Cameroon, along the Ogowe River in Gabon, in Congo and parts of Zaire and Nigeria. Man is infected by the bite of the Chrysops fly carrying infectious larvae.

Clinical picture

These larvae develop into adult *Filariae* that migrate through the human subcutaneous tissue causing migratory swellings typically near joints, so called Calabar swellings (figure 11.4). The adult worms may also appear in the conjunctiva of the eye, the eye worm. Fever is absent, but eosinophilia is prominent. The typical clinical presentation (migratory swellings and/or eye worm in a traveller returning from Gabon) is the key to recognizing loiasis.

Diagnosis, treatment, prevention

Filaria serology is helpful. The identification of microfilariae in blood or body fluids is diagnostic but microfilariae are found in the blood of less than 50% of patients. Diethylcarbamazine which kills both the adults and microfilariae is the treatment of choice. Severe reactions (headache, even encephalitis) may occur; the treatment is started with a low dose that is gradually increased. Normally, corticosteroids are given during the first 3 days of treatment. Surgical removal of the adult worm should be performed whenever possible (14).

Figure 11.4   A, B Calabar swelling of the right hand in a female patient with Loa loa infection

A

B

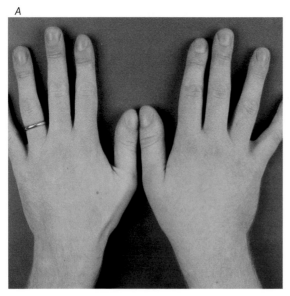
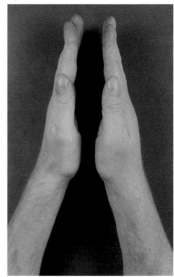

REFERENCES

1   Guzman MG, Kouri G. Dengue: an update. *Lancet Infectious Diseases* 2002;2(1): 33-42.

2   Halstead SB, Streit TG, Lafontant JG, et al. Haiti: absence of dengue hemorrhagic fever despite hyperendemic dengue virus transmission. *Am J Trop Med Hyg* 2001;65(3):180-3.

3   Malavige GN, Fernando S, Fernando DJ, Seneviratne SL. Dengue viral infections. *Postgrad Med J* 2004;80(948):588-601.

4   Mairuhu AT, Wagenaar J, Brandjes DP, van Gorp EC. Dengue: an arthropod-borne disease of global importance. *Eur J Clin Microbiol Infect Dis* 2004;23(6):425-33.

5   Rothman AL. Dengue: defining protective versus pathologic immunity. *Journal of Clinical Investigation* 2004;113(7):946-51.

6   Jensenius M, Fournier PE, Raoult D. Rickettsioses and the international traveler. *Clin Infect Dis* 2004;39(10):1493-9.

7   Rolain JM, Jensenius M, Raoult D. Rickettsial infections – a threat to travellers? *Current Opinion in Infectious Diseases* 2004;17(5):433-7.

8   Zanetti G, Francioli P, Tagan D, Paddock CD, Zaki SR. Imported epidemic typhus. *Lancet* 1998;352(9141):1709.

9   Jensenius M, Fournier PE, Kelly P, Myrvang B, Raoult D. African tick bite fever. *Lancet Infect Dis* 2003;3(9):557-64.

10 Vries PJ de, Kerst JM, Kortbeek LM. Migrerende zwellingen uit Azie: gnathostomiasis. *Ned tijdschr Geneesk* 2001;145(7):322-5.

11 Camacho SPD, Willms K, Otero MDD et al. Acute outbreak of gnathostomiasis in a fishing community in Sinaloa, Mexico. *Parasitology International* 2003;52(2): 133-40.

12 Magana M, Messina M, Bustamante F, Cazarin J. Gnathostomiasis: Clinicopathologic study. *American Journal of Dermatopathology* 2004;26(2):91-5.

13 Kraivichian K, Nuchprayoon S, Sitichalernchai P, Chaicumpa W, Yentakam S. Treatment of cutaneous gnathostomiasis with ivermectin. *American Journal of Tropical Medicine and Hygiene* 2004;71(5):623-8.

14 Case Record 1-2002. *New Engl J Med* 2002;346(2):115-22.

12 *Sexually transmitted infections*

M. Waugh

12.1 INTRODUCTION – DEFINITION

Sexually transmitted infections (STI) are defined as communicable infections passed by sexual routes between human beings. The definition includes most cases of human immunodeficiency virus (HIV) infection. STI cover those infections previously known as venereal disease (VD) and sexually transmitted disease (STD).

World Health Organisation (WHO) 2001 stated that STI are a major global cause of acute illness, infertility, long term disability and death, with severe medical and psychological consequences for millions of men, women and children (1).

WHO estimated that 340 million new cases of curable STI, syphilis, gonorrhoea, chlamydia, and trichomoniasis have occurred throughout the world in 1999 in men and women aged 15-49 years (2). The last year such an estimate was made, was 1999. It was based on previously published similar methodologies in 1990 and 1995. Data for the estimation was based on prevalence and incidence, both in the literature and WHO country files for STI. Estimates from most countries are hampered by the poor quality of prevalence and incidence data. Few studies are community based and the majority of studies have been based in specific populations such as STI or antenatal clinic attendees. Other limitations are small sample sizes, differing diagnostic approaches and study designs used.

STI enhance the sexual transmission of HIV infection. The presence of an untreated STD (ulcerative or non-ulcerative) can increase the risk of acquisition and transmission of HIV by a factor of up to 10. WHO estimated in 2004 that 40 million people in the world were living with HIV. The AIDS epidemic has claimed 3 million lives and 5 million people had acquired HIV in 2004. It is thought that 17 million people are living with HIV in Eastern and Southern Africa, the hardest hit subregion of the world.

There are more than 20 pathogens transmissible through sexual intercourse. STI caused by bacteria are curable with appropriate antimicrobial treatment but they are of major public health concern in industrialised and developing countries and where reportage occurs, the conditions most likely to be reported.

The natural history of STI is such that much of the infection, especially in women, is asymptomatic. Only part of the symptomatic population seeks health care of which most of the cases will in most societies not be reported.

This makes for paucity in case-finding and audit of diagnosis. Report-based STI surveillance systems tend to underestimate the total number of new cases.

In developing countries, STI and their complications are among some of the most frequent categories for which adults seek health care. In women of childbearing age, STI (excluding HIV) are second only to maternal factors as causes of disease, death and healthy life lost.

The highest rates of STI are generally found in urban men and women in their sexually most active years, that is between the ages of 15 and 35. Women tend to become infected at an earlier age than men.

12.2 EPIDEMIOLOGY

STI have always been frequent in large cities especially where large numbers of young adults congregate. In developing countries economic factors and political unrest make for internal migration, such as movement to large cities in India or China; armies moving soldiers long distances away from home territories; or going to work in mining camps in Africa, or Asia. STI s are often spread along long distance transport routes via a combination of lorry drivers and sex workers. The sexual needs of men are supplied by commercial sex- workers often coerced into the trade by poverty, social factors, and drug dependence and kept very often at the work by force by criminals. STI s are the result of sexual liaisons without adequate protection with condoms. Men returning home may infect their wives and sexual partners in the local community. These are factors in the spread of HIV.

Poor education, low economic status, alcohol and street drugs all play roles in STI transmission. In many countries women have little education, little status and very few rights. Yet it is on women that the major burden of STI will fall. It is on women that the main task of child raising will depend. Throughout sub-Saharan Africa there are many orphans, the result of their mothers dying from AIDS (table 12.1).

WHO (2001) calculated the following prevalence and annual incidence of curable (bacterial) STI in adults in 1999.

Table 12.1 Geographical distribution

Region	Population 15-49 (million)	Prevalence (million)	Prevalence per/1000	Annual incidence (million)
North America	156	3	19	14
West Europe	203	4	20	17
North Africa & Middle East	165	3.5	21	10
East Europe & Central Asia	205	6	29	22
Sub-Saharan Africa	269	32	119	69
Southeast Asia	955	48	50	151
East Asia & Pacific	815	6	7	18
Australia & New Zealand	11	0.3	27	1
Latin America & Caribbean	260	18.5	71	38
Total	3040	116.5		340

Estimated prevalence and annual incidence of curable STI by region. Adapted from table 1(2).

The largest number of new infections occurred in South and Southeast Asia, followed by sub-Saharan Africa and Latin America and the Caribbean. However, the highest rate of new cases per 1000 population has occurred in sub-Saharan Africa.

Migration

Migration has always occurred in human societies. In a way, all mankind is descended from immigrants. There are many reasons why an individual or his family migrates. It is known that the male immigrant usually migrates first, his family joining him when he becomes employed. It is at the period when a young male adult is by himself in a strange city be it at home or abroad that he is most likely to contract STI. Then it may also be found that he has contracted syphilis after serologic testing for syphilis or is infected with HIV. STDs more commonly found in the tropics with chronic signs such as lymphogranuloma venereum (LGV) are uncommon, though they may occasionally present at health care centres for migrants.

Imported STI do not need to come from another continent. Movement of young adults takes place all the time within continents or within subcontinents.

Typical examples would be economic migration from eastern to western Europe, and from rural areas to cities in China.

Tourism

The phenomenon of tourists and travellers bringing back STI to their home countries after unsafe sexual intercourse while abroad has its origins in the Grand Tour and military personnel returning from campaigns. Relatively inexpensive fast airflights available to a mass market have allowed for frequent cases of STI found in returning travellers who have not heeded safer sex techniques. Not only will the immediate diagnosis of STD need to be made and treatment started, but local contact tracing may need to be started, should sexual intercourse have also occurred since the return of the patient. Counselling as to risk and HIV testing will need to be done. Some groups run more risks than others.

Homosexual men

The well-travelled homosexual male in western society is particularly at risk to acquiring STI imported from other countries either in his own country or abroad. Examples are the devastating epidemic of AIDS in gay men in North America, Europe and Australasia in the 1980s, resurgent syphilis in Western Europe in the late 1990s after treatment of HIV infection with highly active antiretroviral therapy (HAART) and recent outbreaks of LGV in Western Europe in gay males since 2003.

The last 2 examples are mainly due to unprotected anal sex (bare-back riding).

Acceptable health care needs to be provided for this large group together with information on prevention of STI, condoms, diagnostic and treatment facilities for all STI and easy availability immunisation programmes against hepatitis A and B. Similar facilities which require interpreters with social skills will also need to be provided in large cities in Europe where immigrants congregate. Of course STD treatment centres need to be available for the general population. In many cases facilities may be integrated with pre-existing health care delivery systems.

12.3 MODE OF INFECTION

STI are transmitted by sexual intercourse and other direct contact between an infected and uninfected mucous surface when two people come together intimately.

Several STI may be also transmitted by contaminated blood or blood products. There are more than 25 such diseases. The majority may be passed by penile-vaginal, penile-anal, penile-oral, oral-vaginal, oral-anal sex. Penile-anal and penile-vaginal sex are the means most likely to pass on HIV. Heavy mouth kissing transmits Epstein-Barr virus and cytomegalovirus infection (CMV), both causing glandular fever like illnesses. Scabies and pediculosis pubis may be passed by close body contact with an infected person.

Congenital Infection

Syphilis may be acquired from an untreated mother. Neo-natal CMV infection is similarly acquired. HIV infection if no anti retroviral preventative treatment (HAART) is given in the ante-natal period may passed from maternal blood or the placenta, via the vagina at labour or later via breast feeding. Herpes virus infection mainly type II may be passed on from the vagina if there is a viremia at the time of open delivery causing neo-natal herpes. Genital human papilloma virus (HPV) infections are considered to be a cause of both laryngeal and genital HPV infection in infants. In many parts of the world outside the industrialised countries hepatitis B can be transmitted at birth from a HBsAg positive mother to her child, particularly if she carries e antigen. *Neisseria gonorrhoeae* and *Chlamydia trachomatis* may both be passed from the vagina at delivery, both causing neonatal conjunctivitis and *C. trachomatis* is also thought to cause infection of the naso-pharynx and possibly a neonatal pneumonia.

Familial Spread

Scabies and threadworms may well be spread from an infected person acquired by the sexual mode, to other household contacts.

■ Oral-anal transmission (rimming) and brachio-proctal practices (fisting, fist-fucking).

Any ano-rectal pathogen may be transmitted this way.

■ Infections acquired by the faecal-oral route.

Among others reported are *Escherichia histolytica, E. hartmanni, E. coli, Endolimax nana, Iodamoeba butschlii, Giardia intestinalis, Dientamoeba fragilis,* and *Chilomastix mesnili.*

Cryptosporidium found in HIV infection may well be passed in faecal transmission in sex practices. Nematodes, *Enterobius vermicularis* and *Strongyloides stercoralis* have been found to be transmitted after oro-anal sex. Shigella spp. and Campylobacter spp. and hepatitis A are implicated in transmission this way as well.

■ Infections spread by mucosal/skin contact during anal intercourse.

This includes pathogens well known to cause STI s as well as some less well known.

The list includes *Neisseria gonorrhoea, Neisseria meningitidis, Treponema pallidum,* rectal spirochaetosis, *C. trachomatis,* and possibly *Mycoplasma hominis* and *Ureaplasma urealyticum,* LGV, donovanosis (granuloma inguinale), herpes simplex virus (HSV), hepatitis B virus and CMV and enterovirus 11.

12.4 CLINICAL PICTURE, DIAGNOSTIC PROCEDURES FOR STI

It must be remembered that most are ubiquitous. For simplicity they may be classified as:

- Genital ulceration: syphilis, herpes genitalis, chancroid, LGV, donovanosis (granuloma inguinale).
- Genital discharge: gonorrhoea, Chlamydial infection, bacterial vaginosis (BV), candidosis.
- Superficial: condylomata acuminata (genital human papilloma virus infection), molluscum contagiosum, scabies, pediculosis pubis.
- Systemic: viral – HIV/AIDS, hepatitis A,B,C, Epstein Barr and cytomegalovirus infection. These latter will not be discussed in detail in this text.

12.4.1 Syphilis

Syphilis is an infectious disease caused by *Treponema pallidum*. If it is not treated, it may run a chronic course, systemic from the outset, capable of involving most organs, and able to simulate many other diseases. It is distinguished by florid manifestations and periods of asymptomatic latency. Most cases are venereally acquired but it may be endemic, sporadic, congenital and iatrogenic (3).

Clinical characteristics and course

Primary syphilis
This has an incubation period of 2-6 weeks but may be as long as 3 months. A chancre develops at the point of entry together with regional lymphadenopathy. It may be also in the anal area or mouth.
Diagnosis Provided no antiseptics or treponemicidal antibiotics have been used, from the ano-genital region dark field microscopy will demonstrate *T. pallidum*. This is more difficult to perform than may seem. It is dangerous to do if the patient is HIV positive because of possible blood contamination. Serologic tests for syphilis at this stage may still not be positive.

Secondary Syphilis
This occurs 1-6 months after primary syphilis in an untreated person. A rash, which may take many forms often involving the palms and soles, occurs. Other features are alopecia, mucous patches, condyloma lata, lymphadenopathy, fever, headaches, malaise, hepatitis, nephritis, and arthritis, and sometimes signs of cranial nerve involvement.

Latency divided into disease ensuing-early < 1 year and late > 1 year.

Tertiary Syphilis
Gummata, neurosyphilis and cardiovascular syphilis are rare in modern times.

Diagnosis – serologic tests for syphilis

Specific anti-*T. pallidum* immunoglobulin M (IgM) is detectable in the second week of infection and the production of specific anti-treponemal IgG begins at the fourth week of infection.

Serologic tests. If the Enzyme Immuno-Assay (EIA) (treponemal EIA) is used as a primary screening test, then the Treponema Pallidum Particle (Heamagglutination) Assay TPPA (TPHA) can serve as the confirmatory test. If TPPA (TPHA) is used as a primary screening test EIA can serve as a confirmatory test. For an optimal test TPPA (TPHA) should be quantitative. One should realise that in many parts of the world all that is done are VDRL/RPR (Venereal Disease Research Laboratory / Rapid Plasma Reagine) tests but these may have sensitivity of 100% by the secondary stage.

12.4.2 Herpes genitalis

HSV-1 and HSV-2 are transmitted through direct contact with infected skin lesions, mucous membranes and secretions. Genital herpes is sexually transmitted causing vesicles breaking down to form shallow painful often-recurrent genital ulcers with inguinal lymphadenopathy. It may be primary, recurrent or sub-clinical, caused by reactivation of latent HSV infection in a person without clinically recognised symptoms (4) (figure 12.1). In developed countries its recurrence and infectivity have caused in recent years much medical debate as to its therapy and psychological distress to patients. It has probably been misdiagnosed with chancroid and primary syphilis in many clinical settings around the world. Resistance to acyclovir has been reported in patients who are HIV positive. Pregnant women who contract genital

Figure 12.1   Herpes genitalis: ulceration

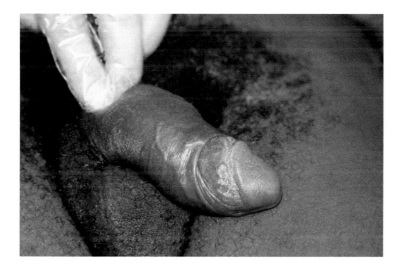

herpes in late pregnancy run a high risk of transmitting the virus to the neonate and should be delivered by Caesarean section.

Diagnostic tests
Viral culture allowing viral amplification and sub typing are the gold standard. Antigen detection tests are useful in that they allow fast confirmation of clinical diagnosis.

12.4.3 Chancroid
This is an acute, ulcerative disease localised to the genitals and often associated with an inguinal bubo (figure 12.2). It is caused by *Haemophilus ducreyi*, a gram-negative facultative anaerobic bacillus that requires haemin (X factor) for growth.

Diagnosis
Actually there is no simple and inexpensive laboratory test available. For this reason in the low resource settings where chancroid is prevalent, the diagnosis is commonly made on clinical grounds alone (5).

12.4.4 Lymphogranuloma venereum
Lymphogranuloma venereum (LGV) is caused by distinct immunotypes of *C. trachomatis*, using micro-immunofluorescence techniques L-1, L-2, L-3.

It has a short incubation period, after which a small transient vesicle appears, at the site of inoculation. Two weeks later the inguinal lymph nodes become large, fluctu-

Figure 12.2   Chancroid

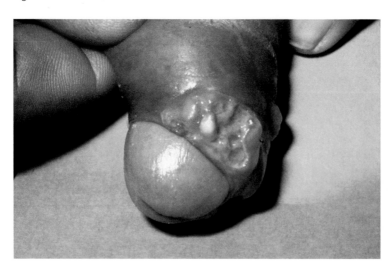

ant and matted together, eventually breaking down and discharging pus. Scarring, fistulae and strictures develop in the ano-genital region. Recently there have been outbreaks in HIV positive homosexual men in Europe presenting with a bloody proctitis.

Diagnosis
Diagnosis is made by referring sera for micro-immunofluorescent techniques, but this is only possible from a few centres.

12.4.5 Granuloma inguinale
Granuloma inguinale (donovanosis) is caused by the intracellular bacterium *Calymmatobacterium granulomatis*. After a variable incubation period of 3 days to 6 months, it causes an itchy papule which breaks down to form a painless but increasingly enlarging genital ulcer. This may rapidly progress into the inguinal regions causing a stinking plaque, which often causes fistula formation.

Diagnosis
Diagnosis is made by biopsy from the edge of the lesion using Leishman, Giemsa, or Wright`s stain. It needs an observer highly skilled in the technique to observe organisms with intense polar staining, resembling closed safety pins within mononuclear leukocytes.

12.4.6 Gonorrhoea
Cause: *Neisseria gonorrhoeae*

Infection of columnar epithelium causes a polymorphonuclear leucocytic response.

This usually causes a purulent urethritis 2-14 days after intercourse be it vaginal, anal or oral with an infected sexual contact. At the time of examination *C. trachomatis* may also be detected if diagnostic facilities allow in up to 60% of cases of gonorrhoea. It should be realised that the often dual etiology of *N. gonorrhoeae* and *C. trachomatis* makes it nigh impossible to describe symptomatology purely to either gonorrhoea or *C. trachomatis* genital infection. Dysuria and the amount of discharge are variable. A few men have hardly any symptoms.

Gonorrhoea in women may be asymptomatic, the woman attending the physician as a sexual contact of a male with gonorrhoea or for some other reason. There may be dysuria or vaginal discharge but the latter may well be due to concomitant *Trichomonas vaginalis*.

On examination, depending on length of infection there may be pus at the urethra and on speculum examination at the cervix.

Acute pelvic inflammatory disease (PID): if there is inflammation of fallopian tubes (acute pelvic inflammatory disease), which occurs in 10% of women with untreated gonorrhoea, there may be a history of lower abdominal pain worse after menstruation. These will be tender on bimanual pelvic examination but laparoscopy shows that abdominal pain may be minimal.

Not only *N. gonorrhoeae* may be a cause of PID but it also has a multifactoral etiology. *Chlamydia trachomatis,* possibly *Mycoplasma hominis* and *Ureaplasma urealyticum* have been isolated from uterine tubes in acute salpingitis.

Rectal gonorrhoea may be asymptomatic or there may be anal discharge or discomfort. Again the patient may attend as a contact or for some other reason. Complications include perianal and ischio-rectal abscesses.

Tonsillar or pharyngeal gonorrhoea may be asymptomatic. Sometimes there may be a pharyngitis.

Figure 12.3 *Gonorrhoea with right epididymo-orchitis*

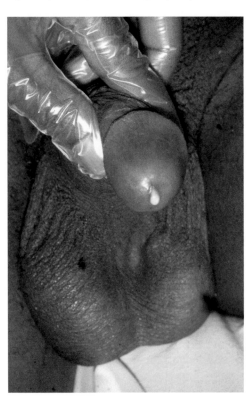

If diagnostic facilities allow it is wise to take cultures for *N. gonorrhoea* from all possible sites of sexual contact.

Adult gonococcal ophthalmia may sometimes occur as a result of infection at coitus. Where hygiene facilities are poor it may be spread then by person to person spread.

Complications

In the male, peri-urethral abscess, epididymo-orchitis (figure 12.3) and an acute prostatitis may occur. In developing countries urethral strictures still occur. A peri-urethral abscess may lead on to fistula.

In the female, Bartholin's gland abscess is a rare complication in industrialised countries being more common where diagnostic facilities are poor. Chronic pelvic inflammatory disease may be asymptomatic until investigation for infertility is started.

The symptoms are variable.

Disseminated gonococcal infection in both sexes: this is more common in women than men. Gonococcal strains associated with disseminated infection have been reported due to serogroupW1 and auxotype AHU– being sensitive to benzylpenicillin.

Usually a fever, skin rash often to begin with haemorrhagic or pustular on an erythematous base, joint pains and a polyarticular arthritis of the knees, wrists, small joints of the hands, ankles, and elbows occur. Alternatively there may be monoarticular arthritis. Diagnosis is made by isolating *N. gonorrhoea* from a lesion or joint fluid.

Gonococcal perihepatitis, meningitis, endocarditis, and pericarditis are rare complications.

Diagnostic procedures

There has been very rapid progress in sophisticated laboratory diagnosis in recent years for most of the pathogens implicated in STI. These are based on polymerase chain reaction (PCR) or serology based on enzyme immunoassay. Office versions applicable to clinical bench diagnosis have been made available. While many of these tests are available in industrialised countries they are not available everywhere. It will be assumed that microscopy may be carried out. Then diagnostic tests will be noted that are main stream and used with success in many centres.

Microscopy

Gram stain of urethral smear-men: 90% pick up; cervix-women: 40-60% pick up, rectal canal-homosexual men: 50% pick up. Hence importance of cultures as well. Gram-negative intracellular diplococci under x 1000 oil immersion suggestive, but not definitive for diagnosis. Methylene blue is sometimes used, but lacks sensitivity and specificity.

Culture

Gold standard but requirements for optimal performance are rigorous (6) – Modified Thayer – Martin or New York City Medium. Because of the rapidly changing patterns of antimicrobial resistance, it is important that there are regional centres for the surveillance of antimicrobial resistance.

12.4.7 Non-gonococcal urethritis(NGU) and Chlamydia trachomatis

These terms are not quite synonymous.

NGU by definition is any urethritis not caused by *N. gonorrhoeae*

This is the commonest form of urethritis in industrialised countries. It is also likely to be as common in developing countries but further studies needed on epidemiology there. *C. trachomatis* is the causative organism of 40 to 60% of NGU. *Mycoplasma genitalium* may play a role.

Clinical Picture

NGU may present with minimal symptoms. There may be a long incubation period of up to 30 days, but some patients notice symptoms within a few days. There is dysuria and urethral discharge, which is variable, sometimes worse in the morning causing a gleet. Recurrence is a common finding.

12.4.8 Chlamydial genital infection

As diagnostic procedures have advanced and as the sexually active public, especially women, seek sexual health check ups, understanding of adult Chlamydial infection has increased.

There may be no symptoms and very few signs in adult males or females, yet *C. trachomatis* may be isolated from relevant sites. There may be variable dysuria and discharge in both sexes. There may be anal discomfort in ano-rectal Chlamydial infection.

Complications

Men: *C. trachomatis* is a common cause of epididymo-orchitis in sexually active men being much more frequent than urinary tract infections in those under 40. Prostatitis may also occur.

Sexually acquired reactive arthritis (SARA) – Reiter's syndrome is likely to occur in non-treated Chlamydial infection in males if they are HLA-B27 positive. It seems less common in industrialised countries with better diagnostic tests than previously. The main signs are circinate balanitis, acute arthritis involving any of the joints, tenosynovitis, palato-buccal lesions, conjunctivitis and later more chronically keratoderma blenorrhagicum, nail changes including onycholysis, sacro-ileitis, and peri-carditis. It is rare in women.

In women PID both acute and chronic, already mentioned as a complication of gonorrhoea, frequently occur. Perihepatitis may also occur,

Diagnostic procedures

Microscopy of urethral smear by gram stain excludes gonorrhoea but shows a poly-morpho nuclear-cytosis with increase of white cells to over 4 per high power field.

C. trachomatis (at present most efficient tests but not available everywhere PCR-nucleic acid amplification tests) may be detected in infected humans from the genital tract, pharynx and ano-rectal canal. PCR techniques have been used also to succes-sfully diagnose using non-invasive methods, urine (both sexes) and self inserted vag-inal tampons and self instructed vulval swabbing.

Tissue culture remains the standard by which other tests are evaluated but sen-sitivity is less than 100%. It still needs to be performed where there may be medico-legal implications such as child sex abuse or rape. Nevertheless PCR techniques have made enormous advances in clinical practice in industrialised countries.

12.4.9 Causes of vaginal discharge

In western countries this is the commonest presenting feature in women.

Bacterial vaginosis (BV) is the commonest vaginal infection in sexually active women. BV may be diagnosed if any 3 of the following criteria are positive, homoge-neous thin discharge, vaginal pH > 4.5, release of a fishy odour due to amines from the vaginal discharge on alkanisation with 10% potassium hydroxide (KOH) and clue cells on wet mount (7). Unlike vaginal infections due to Candida spp. or *Trichomonas vaginalis* there is not usually erythema of the vagina.

Trichomoniasis (TV) is caused by *Trichomonas vaginalis*. It causes a frothy yellow dis-charge with a vulvo-vaginitis. When severe, the cervix has patches of high vascular density described as a strawberry cervix. TV is no longer so common in the West, but much more frequently found in Russia and developing countries in Africa. It is not often found in males as a cause of urethritis but has been reported from Africa.

Diagnosis

Diagnosis made by microscopy and culture, using Feinberg-Whittington medium or newer Elisa tests.

12.4.10 Candidosis

There has been seen in industrialised countries, and in developing countries living on convenience foods and getting obese, an increase in vaginal candidosis and balanoposthitis. Although vaginal discharge is said to cause pruritus, symptoms may be variable.

Diagnosis

Swabs from the anterior fornix in women and glans penis in men are adequate for KOH preparations and direct microscopy, stained smears, and yeast culture based on Sabouraud methodology. Yeast sampling is beyond the scope of this text but is described (8).

12.4.11 STD's on the skin and mucous membranes

Genital warts – condyloma acuminata usually are multiple exophytic and cauliflower-like, growing on the external genitalia of both sexes (figure 12.4). They may also occur around the anus and in the anal canal. Gynaecological and rectal examination may be needed to detect them in hidden sites.

Fig. 12.4   Genital warts in pregnancy

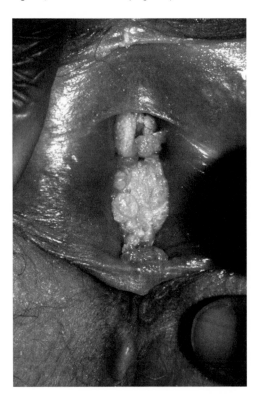

Diagnosis

This is usually made on clinical grounds.

Acetic acid test is useful in diagnosing flat condylomata but it is not highly specific or sensitive for condylomata. However a number of techniques have been introduced which aid in diagnosis. In women colposcopy may be needed to rule out cervical condyloma, dysplasia or neoplasia. Type-specific serological assays are being developed but not yet sensitive enough or type specific. Nucleic acid hybridization techniques have also been developed. These allow for HPV typing but again that is still only used as a highly specialised test.

12.4.12 Molluscum contagiosum

Molluscum contagiosum (MC) is caused by a double stranded DNA poxvirus.

The diagnosis is usually made on clinical examination. It is common in patients in the genital region at STI departments and other STI should be excluded. It may coexist with genital warts.

MC in atypical positions in adults, the flanks, and face should alert to the possibility of co-existent HIV infection.

12.4.13 Scabies

Scabies, this is again commonly found in young sexually active adults and young immigrants living crowded in poor housing without adequate washing facilities. It may be chronic and may have been misdiagnosed as a banal skin condition.

It is important not to miss single lesions on the penis and buttocks and scattered lesions on the lower abdomen. Again the importance of communal treatment to prevent person-to-person spread is stressed.

12.4.14 Pediculosis pubis

Pediculosis pubis, this is often missed until a super infection is noted. In the hirsute male, careful examination needs to be done, not only of the genital region but abdominal, axillary hair and eyelashes.

Nits cemented to the pubic hair are laid at the base as the hair grows, the nit case is found at the distal end of the hair, an aid to how long infection has lasted.

12.5 TREATMENT OF STI

12.5.1 Principles of Treatment

The treatment must be curative where possible. There should be alternatives. It should be easy to administer with few side effects. Where possible it is best given under supervision to make sure of its use or ease of use by the patient. It should be cheap. Not all these criteria are possible.

Sexual partners should be contacted (partner notification) for all STI which are curable or have long term systemic impact. Epidemiological for sexual contacts with bacterial STI should be given.

Care should be taken administering any drug to pregnant women.

Syphilis primary and secondary:
Benzathine penicillin G, 2.4 million IU IM.
Doxycycline 100 mg orally for 15 days.

Gonorrhoea:
Treat as though resistant to penicillin and quinolones.
Cefixime 400 mg stat.
Ceftriaxone 250 mg IM.
Spectinomycin 2 g IM.

Many clinicians also treat for *C. trachomatis* at the same time.

Chlamydial infection and NGU:
Doxycycline 100 mg bd for 7 days.
Azithromycin 1g stat.
Oxytetracycline 500 mg qid for 7 days.
Ofloxacin 200 mg bd for 7 days.

Chancroid:
Erythromycin 500 mg qid for 7 days.
Azithromycin 1g stat.
Ceftriaxone 250 mg IM.

LGV:
Doxycycline 100 mg bd,
Erythromycin 500 mg qid,
Tetracycline 500 mg qid, all for 21 days.

Granuloma inguinale:
Azithromycin 500 mg daily for 7 days.
Or 1g weekly for 4 weeks.
Doxycline 100 mg bd for 21 days.
Erythromycin 800 mg po bd for 21 days.

Genital herpes:
Antiviral therapy reduces shedding, and when used prophylactically reduces rate of recurrences.
Acyclovir 200 mg 5 times a day for 5 to 10 days for primary attacks or episodic therapy.
Recurrent suppressive therapy 400 mg bd for 6 months.

Genital warts:
Ablation, electro-cautery, cryo-therapy.
Podophyllotoxin solution or cream applied by patient bd for 3 days, may be repeated up to 4 weeks, not to be used in pregnancy.
Imiquimod apply up to 3 times a week till lesions go, max. 16 weeks.
Both local treatments may cause erythema.

Molluscum contagiosum:
Destroy each lesion with needle or comedo extractor, cryo-therapy.

Scabies and pediculosis pubis:
Permethrin and malathion preparations as per makers' instructions.
In some places where water is scarce, ivermectin 200 µg/kg by mouth in one dose with care.

Candidosis:
Imidazoles, clotrimazole, econazole, miconazole fluconazole, itraconazole topically, vaginal tablets or in some case orally effective.
Nystatin pessary at nights for 14 days effective.

Trichomoniasis:
Metronidazole 2 g stat (5 x 400 mg), or 200 mg bd for 7 days also given to the male.
Should not be given in first trimester of pregnancy. Resistant cases are seen.

Bacterial vaginosis:
Metronidazole 2 g stat or 400 mg bd for 7 days.

12.6 **PREVENTION**

Immunisation

Hepatitis A and hepatitis B should be offered to any individual who is not immune in whom it is perceived they are at risk to these infections sexually or through being a contact of drug abusers.

At the present no other effective vaccines are available. Vaccine against HPV is being developed.

Education, empowerment, integrated and continuing about STI, needs to start from childhood, continued into adolescence and throughout sexually active years.

The dangers to the person's own health need to be pointed out in a way that is understood. The effects on others and the possibility of sterility, and early death in AIDS need to be emphasised.

Condom use needs promotion and there needs to be ease in obtaining them.

In many culture the need to let women make their own decisions, at present denied to them needs political good will.

The individual needs to have always adequate and up to date information.

This may be found on the Internet http://www.unaids.org

REFERENCES

1   World Health Organisation. Geneva, 2001:WHO/CDS/CSR/EDC/2001.10

2   World Health Organisation Global Prevalence and Incidence of Selected Curable Sexually Transmitted Infections Overview and Estimates. WHO/HIV_AIDS/2001.02

3   Waugh MA. Syphilis. In: Katsambas AD, Lotti TM. European Handbook of Dermatological Treatments 2nd ed. Berlin: Springer 2003: 512-8.

4   Kroon S. Herpes Genitalis. In: Katsambas AD, Lotti TM European Handbook of Dermatological Treatments 2nd ed. Berlin: Springer 2003:187-92.

5   Eichmann A. Chancroid. In: Elsner P, Eichmann A (eds). Sexually Transmitted Diseases Advances in Diagnosis and Treatment. Basel: Karger 1996:20-4.

6   Lind I, Gonorrhoea. In: Elsner P, Eichmann A (eds). Sexually Transmitted Diseases Advances in Diagnosis and Treatment. Basel: Karger 1996:12-9.

7   Amsel R, Totten PA, Spiegel CA, Chen KCS, Eschenbach DA, Holmes KK. Nonspecific vaginitis: diagnostic criteria and microbial and epidemiologic associations. *Am J Med* 1983;74:14-22.

8   Stary A. Genital Candidosis. In: Elsner P, Eichmann A (eds.). Sexually Transmitted Diseases Advances in Diagnosis and Treatment. Basel: Karger 1996:40-9.

13 Endemic treponematoses

H.J.H. Engelkens

13.1 INTRODUCTION

Treponemal diseases still are widespread. Treponematoses occurring in humans comprise the endemic non-venereal treponematoses (yaws, pinta, and endemic syphilis), and venereal syphilis. These diseases share prominent cutaneous manifestations and a chronic relapsing course. At present the causative agents of the different treponematoses cannot be distinguished from each other serologically or by other means. Venereal syphilis, caused by *Treponema pallidum* subspecies *pallidum* has a completely different mode of transmission, epidemiology, and clinical presentation (see chapter 12). Children are at the highest risk to acquire the non-venereal treponematoses (table 13.1), where sexual transmission does not play a pathogenetic role. Transmission occurs by skin and mucous membrane contact from person to person. In yaws, breaks in the skin provide an entry for the treponemes. Endemic syphilis is most probably transmitted directly or indirectly by skin-to-skin or mouth-to-mouth contacts with infectious lesions, and by contaminated fingers. The mode of transmission of pinta is not entirely clear, probably by direct skin or mucous membrane contact (1,2,3,4).

Table 13.1   Non-venereal endemic treponematoses

Yaws	
(framboesia tropica, bouba, pian, frambesia, parangi, paru)	*Treponema pallidum subspecies pertenue (T. pertenue)*
Endemic syphilis	
(bejel, frangi, njovera, loath, firjal, dichuchwa, bishel)	*Treponema pallidum subspecies endemicum (T. endemicum)*
Pinta	
(carate, azul, cute, mal del pinto, cativa)	*Treponema carateum (T. carateum)*

Mass treatment campaigns against the endemic treponematoses, were very successful in the 1950s and 1960s, with support from the World Health Organization (WHO) and the United Nations Children's Fund (UNICEF). The incidence of the endemic treponematoses has been greatly reduced. Unfortunately, eradication was not accomplished. Precise figures on the current prevalence of endemic treponematoses are rare. There is considerable underreporting. Lack of public health surveillance and prophylactic control measures have resulted in a resurgence of especially yaws in several tropical regions of the world, among people living in unhygienic circumstances in remote, often inaccessible regions. Latent cases are still highly prevalent and millions of people continue to be at risk of acquiring the endemic treponematoses (5,6,7).

Yaws nowadays is prevalent in Africa and Southeast Asia in rural warm tropical regions with high humidity. Endemic syphilis still exists among isolated closed communities under unhygienic, primitive conditions, under dry, arid circumstances in the Eastern hemisphere, among nomads and seminomads in Saudi Arabia and in Sahel countries in Africa. Pinta is still prevalent in tropical Central and South America in remote rural regions (6,8,9).

Figure 13.1 Early yaws. A crustopapillomatous lesion on the arm.

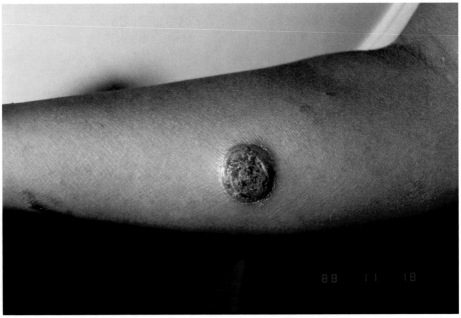

13.2 CLINICAL PICTURE

In endemic treponematoses, an early (infectious) and late (non-infectious) stage are discerned. Most often four stages have been discerned (a primary, secondary, tertiary, and latent stage), like in venereal syphilis. Different stages may show overlapping (1,2,3,4).

In contrast to venereal syphilis, in yaws, pinta and endemic syphilis, congenital infection and neurologic and cardiovascular involvement are assumed to be absent or extremely rare.

Yaws and endemic syphilis may nowadays present an atypical form or a milder, 'attenuated' form in some regions, with less florid skin lesions, especially in areas

Figure 13.2   Multiple lesions on the lower extremities, early yaws

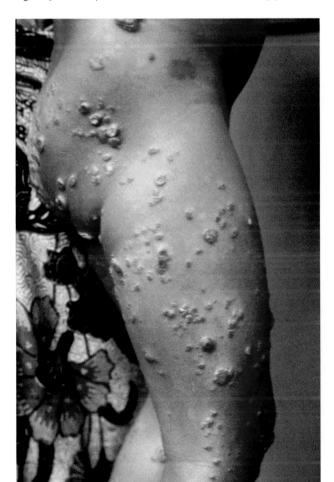

with a low prevalence, possibly by the widespread use of antibiotics, by improvement of social conditions, by a mutation or an adaptation of the causative organism, or by altered immune responses of the host. In HIV-infected patients, new problems with the diagnosis and treatment of sexually transmitted syphilis are described. Thusfar, these problems have not yet been reported in endemic treponematoses; endemic treponematoses occur 'where the highways end', in regions where HIV infection has not yet been introduced (7).

13.2.1 Yaws

The first (early stage) lesion, 'mother yaw' (figure 13.1), appears after an incubation period of 9-90 days. Legs, feet and buttocks are most often affected.

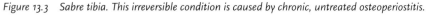

Figure 13.3   Sabre tibia. This irreversible condition is caused by chronic, untreated osteoperiostitis.

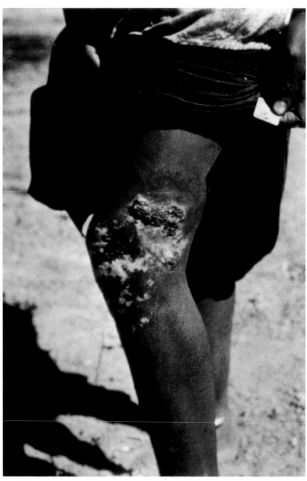

Sometimes, instead of a solitary primary lesion, multiple primary lesions occur. Early stage lesions can develop into ulcerated papillomatous lesions, which are highly infectious. After or during spontaneous disappearance of initial lesions relapses of more disseminated lesions can occur, which may be preceded or accompanied by fever, malaise, headache and generalized lymphadenopathy. These early (secondary) stage skin lesions (figure 13.2) often resemble the 'mother yaw'. Macules, papules and nodules can also be seen. Palms of the hands and soles of the feet may show hyperkeratosis (crab yaws).

Hyperkeratotic lesions can occur in both early and late yaws. In the early stage bone and joint manifestations can already occur. Most important are osteitis and periostitis. After the early skin manifestations have subsided, a latent period of variable duration follows. This period can be interrupted by one or more relapses of skin lesions. In the majority of patients, latency lasts lifelong.

The destructive late stage develops in approximately ten percent of patients. Irreversible lesions of skin, bone and joints are notorious (gangosa, sabre tibia (figure 13.3), gondou) (1,2,3,4).

13.2.2 Endemic syphilis

The primary lesion frequently remains unobserved in endemic syphilis, since the oropharyngeal mucosa is often involved in the primary phase. The first presentation

Figure 13.4   Axillary condylomata of early endemic syphilis. Identical lesions are common in yaws.

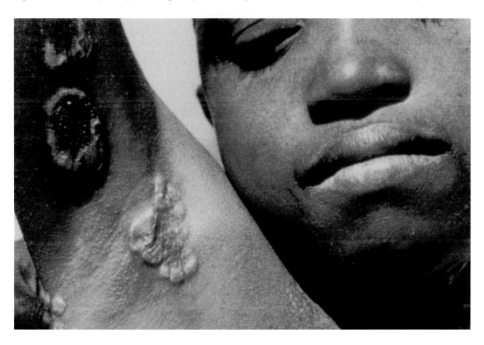

of the disease frequently is a small ulcer or papule on the mucous membranes, non-itchy skin eruptions and generalized lymphadenopathy, resembling yaws or sexually transmitted syphilis. Anogenital or axillary (figure 13.4) condylomata lata, compara-ble to those in yaws and sexually transmitted syphilis, occur.

In the late stage, affection of skin, bones, joints and nasopharynx may lead to severe destruction (1,2,3,4).

13.2.3 Pinta

In the early stage of pinta, a papule or an erythematosquamous plaque (figure 13.5) occurs usually on the legs, feet or hands. The initial lesions may become pigmen-

Figure 13.5   Violaceous psoriatic plaque of early pinta

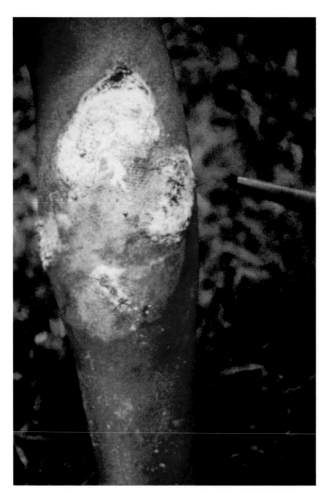

ted, hyperkeratotic and scaly, accompanied by local lymphadenopathy. After several months or even years more extensive skin lesions may appear. Changes in skin pigmentation can be the result of these skin lesions.

In late (tertiary) pinta disfiguring pigmentary changes, achromia, skin atrophy and hyperkeratoses are the main features (figure 13.6). Pinta is considered the most benign of the endemic treponematoses: no mutilations occur. It is assumed that only the skin is affected in this chronic disease (1,2,3,4).

13.3 LABORATORY TESTS

A diagnosis of endemic treponematoses is based on clinical, geographic, epidemiologic and laboratory findings. No serologic test can distinguish between the different treponematoses. Serologic tests for endemic treponematoses are identical to those of venereal syphilis. In use are specific treponemal tests, such as the Treponema pallidum hemagglutination assay (TPHA) and the fluorescent treponemal antibody absorption (FTA-ABS) test, and non-treponemal tests such as the venereal disease research laboratory (VDRL) test and the rapid plasma reagin (RPR) test. The pattern of reactivity after infection and the persistence of positive serological test results after treatment are similar in non-venereal and venereal treponematoses. Positive serological test results (in all stages except the very early stage), the presence of treponemes

Figure 13.6   Hyperpigmented, atrophic skin of late pinta

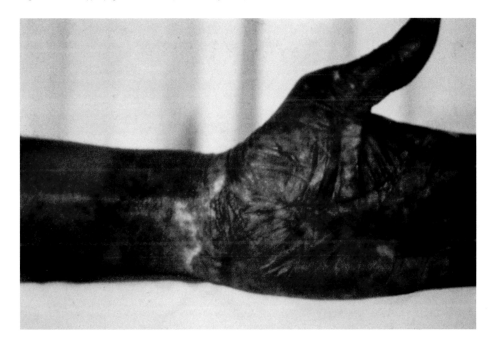

in dark-field examination of exudates of cutaneous lesions and examination of skin biopsies (figure 13.7) confirm the diagnosis.

Available genetic evidence indicates that *T. pallidum* and *T. pertenue* are indistinguishable. However, in a recent study it has been shown that *T. pertenue* and *T. pallidum* differ in at least one nucleotide in a homologous antigen. Further research will hopefully lead to the development of specific tests to differentiate between the treponematoses (10).

13.4 TREATMENT

The current recommended treatment is: a single intramuscular injection of benzathine penicillin 1.2 million U (0.6 million U for children younger than 10 years old) for all patients and contacts (1). Family members, contacts of patients and patients with latent infection should receive the same doses as those suffering from active disease. No resistance to penicillin has as yet been reported. For penicillin-allergic persons, tetracyclins and erythromycin are alternatives.

13.5 CONCLUSION

It is highly unlikely that the different treponematoses will be eradicated. During relapsing infectious periods, persons with latent infection will periodically present with infectious lesions. All contacts exposed are at risk of contracting the disease (1).

Figure 13.7   Numerous treponemes (skin biopsy, Steiner staining method)

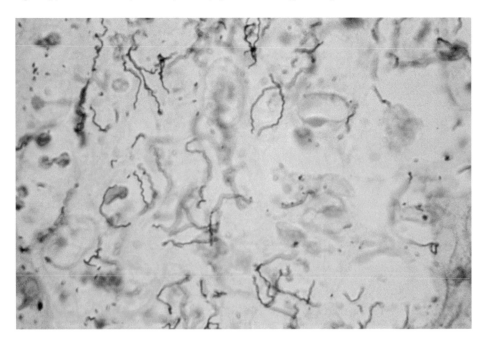

After the mass treatment campaigns of the past, the clinical picture of yaws and endemic syphilis has changed in some regions, with milder attenuated atypical disease, making a proper diagnosis more difficult. Patients do not develop lifelong immunity. Therefore, early detection and treatment campaigns remain crucial. Continuing surveillance by seroepidemiological evaluation remains urgently needed. As is known from the past, treatment campaigns, continuing health education, improvement of social and medical conditions are of utmost importance (1,6,8,9). Eradication programs should be integrated into other existing health programs, for instance vaccination programs, mother and child health clinics, tuberculosis and leprosy programs. Together with existing primary health care services these measures will certainly offer new possibilities to interfere with the spread of the treponematoses.

Due to the increasing frequency of worldwide travel and trends in migration, yaws, endemic syphilis or pinta can turn up anywhere in the world and confront the medical profession with a diagnostic dilemma, especially in latent stage or late stage disease. In a patient originating from an endemic region a positive treponemal serology must arouse suspicion of a non-sexually transmitted treponematosis (1,2,3,4). Shared antigens give rise to cross-reactive antibodies common to all treponemal diseases, thus so far precluding a differential diagnosis on the basis of serologic tests. A careful history and evaluation in patients from endemic regions is still of utmost importance. It remains a mystery whether the above-mentioned causative agents are really different microorganisms (1).

After proper treatment, early infectious lesions of yaws and endemic syphilis heal within two weeks. Healing of the cutaneous lesions of early pinta takes more time. Recognition and treatment of patients suffering from endemic treponematoses in an early stage can prevent later-stage sequels. Without institution of therapy, late stage manifestations can lead to severe handicaps (1,2,3,4,9).

REFERENCES

1   Perine PL, Hopkins DR, Niemel PLA, St.John RK, Causse G, Antal GM. Handbook of Endemic Treponematoses. Yaws, Endemic Syphilis and Pinta. Geneva: World Health Organization, Geneva: 1984.

2   Engelkens HJH, Jubianto Judanarso, Oranje AP, Vuzevski VD, Niemel PL, van der Sluis JJ, Stolz E. Endemic Treponematoses. Part I. Yaws. *Int J Dermatol* 1991;30:77-83.

3   Engelkens HJH, Niemel PLA, Sluis JJ van der, Stolz E. Endemic Treponematoses. Part II. Pinta and endemic syphilis. *Int J Dermatol* 1991;30:231-8.

4   Koff AB, Rosen T. Nonvenereal treponematoses: yaws, endemic syphilis and pinta. *J Am Acad Dermatol* 1993;29:519-37.

5   Endemic treponematoses in the 1980s (editorial). *Lancet* 1983;ii:551-2.

6   Luger A, Meheus A. Drastische ausbreitung endemischer treponematosen. Alarming spread of endemic treponematoses. *Z Hautkr* 1988;63:463-4.

7   Engelkens HJH, Niemel PLA, Sluis JJ van der, Stolz E. The resurgence of yaws. World-wide consequences. *Int J Dermatol* 1991;30:99-101.

8   Programme for the control of the endemic treponematoses. World Health Organization. VDT/EXBUD/87.1; August 1987.

9   Engelkens HJH, Vuzevski VD, Stolz E. Nonvenereal treponematoses in tropical countries. *Clinics Dermatol* 1999;17:143-52.

10 Noordhoek GT. Syphilis and yaws. A molecular study to detect and differentiate pathogenic treponemes. Thesis University of Utrecht, The Netherlands 1991.

14 American cutaneous leishmaniasis

S. Talhari, C. Chrusckiak Talhari, J.A. de Oliveira Guerra

14.1 INTRODUCTION

American cutaneous leishmaniasis (ACL), also known as espundia, pian bois, uta, chiclero's ulcer, bush yaws and other local names, is an infeccious disease caused by different protozoan parasites belonging to the genus Leishmania. The disease is endemic in many countries of Central and South America, presenting a variable clinical spectrum. Leishmaniasis represents an increasing health problem in the world mainly because of new settlements in endemic areas, the opening of new roads in forest zones, tourism and the movement of new immigrants into endemic areas.

14.2 EPIDEMIOLOGY

The worldwide prevalence of leishmaniasis including the visceral form of the disease is about 12 million. According to the World Health Organization (WHO), each year, approximately 500 000 new cases of cutaneous leishmaniasis are diagnosed all around the world, and 300 million people are exposed to the infection [1,2]. Brazil is one of the most endemic countries in the Americas. According to the Brazilian Ministry of Health a total of 22 590 cases were diagnosed in 2004. In the Brazilian Amazon basin, an increasing number of patients has been observed [3,4]. Just in the capital of the federal state of Amazonas, Manaus, a total number of 873 cases was reported in 2004.

ACL is endemic throughout Central and South America It was regarded mainly as an occupational disease, affecting people working in tropical forested areas where they are exposed to the natural transmission cycle of the disease. However, changes in these environments have led to the proliferation of various species of the vector, their associated parasites, and reservoirs around rural settlements [5]. Furthermore, there is an increasing number of reports concerning the presence of vectors and infection in peri-urban zones, which were not previously endemic areas.

Table 14.1   Etiological agents of American cutaneous leishmaniasis

Subgenus Viannia	Subgenus Leishmania
L. (V.) braziliensis	*L. (L.) mexicana*
L. (V.) peruviana	*L. (L.) pifanoi*
L. (V.) guyanensis	*L. (L.) amazonensis*
L. (V.) panamensis	*L. (L.) garnhami*
L. (V.) lainsoni	*L. (L.) venezuelensis*
L. (V.) naiffi	
L. (V.) colombiensis	
L. (V.) shawi	
L. (V.) lindergergi	

14.3 ETIOLOGY AND PATHOGENESIS

ACL is caused by the neotropical *Leishmania* species classified in the subgenera *Viannia* and *Leishmania* (table 14.1).

The vectors of leishmaniasis are phlebotomines belonging to the genus *Lutzomya* and *Psychodopygus*. Phlebotomines are small mosquito-like insects that inoculate the parasite into the skin while taking a blood meal and are widely disseminated throughout the tropical and subtropical regions. Only the females are hematophagous. Generaly, the infection is zoonotic. One species of *Leishmania* may be associated with one, or many domestic and wild vertebrate reservoirs. Humans are commonly accidental hosts, although there are situations in which they may be the reservoir in an anthroponotic cycle (6).

During their life cycle, *Leishmania* species are found in two morphologic forms – amastigotes and promastigotes. In humans and other mammalian hosts, they exist within macrophages as round to oval nonflagellated amastigotes, 2 to 3 μm in diameter. In the arthropod vectors, the parasites exist as elongated flagellated promastigotes, 10 to 15 μm in length and 2 to 3 μm in width. Leishmania are intracellular organisms that primarily infect the macrophages and dendritic cells (DC). After deposition of the promastigotes by the female sandfly vector in the mammalian host, these flagellated forms are taken up by the macrophages and DCs, where they change to and replicate as amastigotes. After several asexual divisions, the amastigotes rupture the cell and are released. They are then rapidly taken up by other macrophages. Some parasites may remain in the skin causing cutaneous lesions, while others can spread from the skin via lymphatics and the blood stream within some weeks after the infection. Parasites may then localize in the nasal, buccal and pharyngeal mucosa leading to mucocutaneous ulcerative lesions in predisposed hosts. The life cycle is completed when the vector ingests the amastigotes from the reservoirs (humans are rare), which then undergo a transformation back to the promastigote form and multiply. Once the promastigotes are fully developed, they migrate from the vector's midgut to the pharynx and proboscis, where they remain until they are inoculated into a new mammalian host.

14.4 IMMUNOLOGIC RESPONSE

After human infection with *Leishmania* parasites, the individuals will develop different degrees of susceptibility to infection, with a wide spectrum of clinical manifestations, or no disease (7,8). Like leprosy, leishmaniasis is considered a spectral disease by some authors.

The immune mechanisms of *Leishmania* infection are dependent on the host immune response. In general lines, cellular mediated immunity plays a major role in the resistance to infection with *Leishmania*. This type of immune reaction is also considered to be crucial for healing of the lesions and development of long-lasting immunity. Infections that are not totally controlled by cellular mediated immunity may evolve to one of two polar forms of the disease, either to the hypersensitivity pole, represented by mucocutaneous leishmaniasis or to the anergic diffuse cutaneous form of the disease, which is associated with the hyposensitivity pole. Mucocutaneous leishmaniasis is considered to be the hypersensitivity pole because in this variant of the disease the antigen is able to stimulate an exaggerated immune response, which continues even though most of the parasites are eliminated. This continuing inflammatory response can cause severe local reactions including the destruction of mucosal and cutaneous tissues. In contrast, in the hyposensivity pole, the patients present a deficient cell-mediated immune response against the leishmanial parasite.

The best known experimental model of leishmaniasis is the infection with *Leishmania major*, one of the etiologic species of the Old World leishmaniasis. In this murine model, while susceptibility and progression of the disease are associated with CD4+ T-helper 2 (Th2) response, which induces the production of interleukin (IL) 4, IL-5, IL-10 and transforming growth factor β, the control and resolution of the infection is related to Th1 response. The secretion of interferon (IFN) γ and IL-2 by Th1 cells also plays an important role in determining resistence to leishmanial infection. Although the elimination of the parasites occurs through an effector mechanism involving an IFN-γ mediated-activation of infected macrophages in the murine model of the disease, the operative mechanism in humans is still not clear (9,10).

In comparison to cell-mediated response, humoral immunity is not correlated with the resolution of the disease.

Most patients do not develop protective lifelong-immunity after infection. Although different types of vaccines are being investigated, such as killed or attenuated whole parasites, synthetic or recombinant peptides, or recombinant live vaccine vectors, an effective vaccine for the prevention of leishmaniasis is still not available.

14.5 **CLINICAL FEATURES**

According to the species of the infecting Leishmania and the patient's cell-mediated immune response, a spectrum of clinical forms of the disease can develop (11,12), including localized cutaneous leishmaniasis (LCL), mucocutaneous leishmaniasis (MCL), and anergic diffuse cutaneous leishmaniasis (ADCL). Moreover, Silveira et al (7) and Turetz et al (13) have added a new clinical feature to this spectrum, a form that his group had called borderline disseminated cutaneous leishmaniasis (BDCL).

Figure 14.1   Cutaneous leishmaniasis Tropical ulcer like.

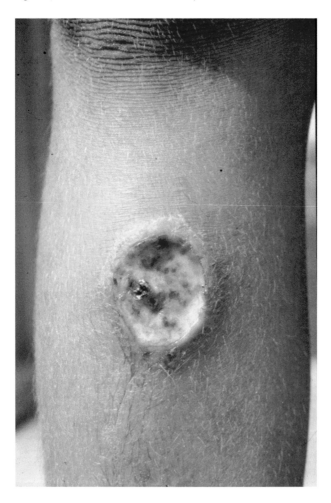

14.5.1 Localized cutaneous leishmaniasis

LCL is the most frequent form of the disease. The disease becomes clinically apparent after a variable incubation period. Clinically, LCL may present as a single or multiple deep ulcerated skin lesions with raised, indurated edges and a sloughy base affecting any exposed parts of the body (figures 14.1 and 14.2). In Mexico and Central America, the lesions localized on the pinna of the ears is called chiclero's ulcer. The lesions can also show a verrucous, vegetative aspect or appear as papules, nodules and infiltrative lesions. There may be satellite lesions, an invasion of proximal lymphatic vessels, which sometimes give a sporotrichoid aspect, and local lymphadenopathy. Therefore, leishmanial parasites can invade the mucous membranes of the mouth,

Figure 14.2 Cutaneous leishmaniasis. Pyoderma like. Children are frequently affected.

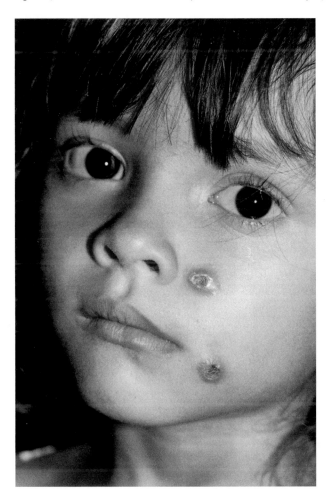

nose, pharynx, and larynx, giving rise to the mucocutaneous forms of the disease. In some patients, the lesions may evolve to spontaneous self-healing over months to years, leaving atrophic scars. Nevertheless, most of the cases require systemic treatment to end the disease and prevent subsequent mucocutaneous involvement.

The causative agent of LCL can be any member of the neotropical subgenera *Viannia* and *Leishmania*. The most important parasite associated with this form of disease is *L. (V.) braziliensis*.

14.5.2 Mucocutaneous leishmaniasis

A small number of patients may simultaneously present skin and metastatic mucosal involvement. However, the majority of patients show MCL as a result of an old, prolonged, untreated or mistreated, and usually self-healing ulcerated skin lesion (figure 14.3).

The time between the disappearance of the skin lesion and development of the mucosal involvement is variable, ranging from 2 to 35 years (average of 10 years). Clinically, the lesions are characterized by the involvement of the nasal mucosa in almost all cases, and in one-third of the patients a second site is affected, usually the

Figure 14.3   A, B Mucocutaneous leishmaniasis. Partial destruction of the nose. Atrophic scar after treatment.

A

B

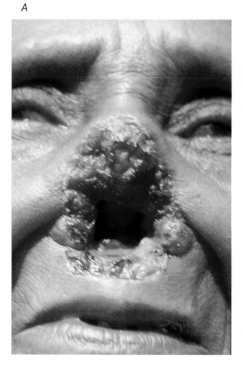
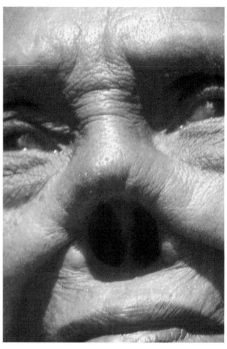

pharynx, palate, larynx or upper lip. The patients generally complain of permanent nasal stuffiness and obstruction, usually showing on physical examination an ulcerated cartilaginous mucosa or a nodule on the inferior turbinate or septum. Granulomas may also be posteriorly located requiring nasendoscopy to be seen. The main pathological feature is necrosis of the nasopharyngeal mucous tissues, which can lead to perforation of the septum and later complete destruction of the nose, palate and lips, causing palatal dysfunction, dysphagia, dysphonia, aspiration and severe disfigurement. The latter clinical feature is known as espundia in South America. Ultimately, death can occur due to secondary infection and/or laryngeal obstruction leading to acute respiratory failure or starvation. Spontaneous healing of MCL is unknown.

The most frequent etiologic agent of this clinical form of leishmaniasis is *L. (V.) braziliensis*, but a smaller proportion of the cases is caused by *L. (V.) panamensis* and *L. (V.) guyanensis*.

14.5.3 Anergic diffuse cutaneous leishmaniasis

In 1946, this rare form of ADCL was described in Venezuela by Convit and Lapenta. Similar cases from other South American countries and also Central and North Americas were subsequently reported. According to the first description, ADCL is characterized by the presence of nodular skin lesions, plaques, ulcerations in areas submitted to trauma and infiltrative disseminated cutaneous lesions distributed over the whole body. The disease also presents a negative Montenegro cutaneous-test and failure to respond to antimonials and other specific therapies. The disease shows a close clinical resemblance to lepromatous leprosy. Although ADCL usually presents a protracted course, there is no tendency to visceralization. The Montenegro skin test and lymphocyte proliferation assay are negative, which demonstrate the deficient cell-mediated immune response characteristic of this form of the disease. The causative agents of ADCL are *L. (L.) pifanoi*, *L. (L.) mexicana* and *L. (L.) amazonensis*.

ADCL in Brazil is predominantly caused by *L. (L.) amazonensis*. The involvement of nasopharyngeal mucous membrane is rare.

14.5.4 Borderline disseminated cutaneous leishmaniasis

Silveira (7) and Turetz (13) reported a new clinical form of leishmaniasis characterized by a relatively rapid dissemination of cutaneous lesions. Moreover, the patients could present simultaneous skin and nasopharyngeal involvement in cases of delayed and untreated evolution. Hundreds of erythematous papules and/or ulcerated skin lesions may appear after two or three months, making it possible to determine the location of the primary and secondary lesions. The concomitant cutaneous and mucosal involvement indicates that active skin infections may persist for long periods and that, in these cases, mucosal lesions therefore represent the final result of infection. *L. (V.) braziliensis* and other species of the subgenus *Viannia* are the most important etiologic agents involved.

The delayed hypersensitivity skin-test reaction to *Leishmania* antigen and the lymphocyte proliferation assays are usually negative during the dissemination of the parasites, which reflects some inhibition of the cell-mediated immune mechanisms in cases of BDCL. This 'incomplete failure' of the cellular immune response in controlling the infection has lead to the term 'borderline'.

14.6 DIFFERENTIAL DIAGNOSIS

Skin lesions that can mimic LCL include traumatic ulcerative lesions, superinfected insect bites, myiasis, fungal and mycobacterial infections, sarcoidosis, neoplasms and many other skin diseases.

The following diseases should be considered in the differential diagnosis of MCL: venereal syphilis, yaws, rhinoscleroma and blastomycosis.

ADCL should be differentiated from lepromatous leprosy.

14.7 DIAGNOSIS

The diagnosis of ACL is based on the presence of the parasites in tissues. The most effective method is a skin smear from the lesion. The smears are obtained by performing a shallow slit in the skin from the edge of the ulcer with a no. 11 blade and staining with Wright's, Giemsa or Leishman. On light microscopy, the amastigotes are seen as pale-blue oval bodies presenting a dark-blue nucleus and a small point-shaped kinetoplast within the cytoplasm of tissue macrophages (figure 14.4).

Alternatively, the parasites can be cultured in a biphasic medium, such as Novy-MacNeal-Nicole (NNN), or a similar medium. Although cultures should not be discarded as negative before 4 weeks, some strains will not grow in culture. In these cases, the material can be inoculated into susceptible animals, such as hamsters. However, it may take 7 to 9 months to give a result, being therefore, a method which is not very practical for routine diagnosis.

Figure 14.4   Leishmaniasis. Positive skin smear: amastigotes inside a tissue macrophage.

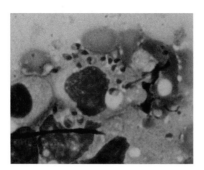

Although the histopathology of the cutaneous lesions is highly variable, ranging from ulceration to hyperplasia, the histopathological examination is still an important diagnostic tool. Generally, light microscopy shows diffuse dermal infiltrate containing histiocytes, lymphocytes, plasma cells and neutrophils. The number of parasites is usually inversely proportional to the duration of the lesion. LCL lesions due to *Viannia* species demonstrate scarce parasites and usually, a mild infiltrate consisting of few macrophages and frequent lymphocytes and plasma cells, which gives the infiltrate characteristics of an epitheliod granuloma. On another hand, localized lesions due to *L. (L.) amazonensis* reveal a heavy dermal infiltrate of vacuolated macrophages full of amastigotes, which gives the infiltrate a macrophagic granuloma appearance. Mucocutaneous lesions may also present granulomatous changes, *Leishmania* parasites are difficult to detect. ADCL lesions are characterized by a dense infiltrate of macrophages presenting abundant amastigotes. There are scarce lymphocytes and plasma cells, giving the infiltrate an aspect of a macrophagic granuloma. In cases of BDCL, the histopathological examination reveals an infiltrate of lymphocytes and plasma cells in the dermis, with rare macrophages and parasites.

Compared to the above mentioned diagnostic methods, the polymerase chain reaction (PCR) is the best approach to diagnose ACL (14). Aside from being highly sensitive and specific, it is also more rapid than the other methods currently available. There are primers to identify different parasite species. As the characterization of parasites may influence the treatment, PCR should be used as a routine examination, especially where cutaneous leishmaniasis is endemic and caused by different parasites. Unfortunately, this very sensitive method is still expensive and not available in most of the endemic areas.

Tests of immune function are available, but are more valuable for following the course of the disease than for diagnosing it. They include enzyme-linked immunosorbent assays (ELISA), the Montenegro test and in vitro lymphocyte proliferation assay for cell-mediated immunity. The ELISA test uses purified leishmanial antigens, showing elevated antibody levels usually in the early stages of the disease. In our experience, it is a very good test to follow the patients with mucocutaneous leishmaniasis after the treatment. The Montenegro skin test, also known as leishmanin test, is used to measure the cell-mediated immune response by injecting 0.1 ml of a phenol-killed preparation of promastigotes in the anterior aspect of the forearm. After 48-72h, the reaction is measured and an induration of 5 mm or more is considered positive. The lymphocyte proliferation assay also evaluates the cell-mediated immune response by measuring the proliferation of peripheral blood lymphocytes in response to a crude extract of promastigotes after a 6-day period of incubation. The Montenegro skin test and lymphocyte proliferation assay indicate both present and past infection.

14.8 **PROPHYLAXIS**

Since there is still no available vaccine against leishmaniasis, measures to combat the vectors should be employed. The increasing incidence and domesticity of ACL reservoirs and vectors, also increase the feasibility of interventions to interrupt transmission around houses. Residual spraying of houses can reduce the transmission through the interruption of leishmanial life-cycle (15,16).

14.9 **TREATMENT**

The drugs of choice for the treatment of ACL are the meglumine antimonate (Glucantime®) and sodium stiboglunate (Pentostam®), both pentavalent antimony derivatives. Amphotericin B and pentamidin are the second-line treatments (17,18).

The recommended dose for localized and disseminated cutaneous leishmaniasis in Brazil is 10-20 mg/kg/day, intravenously or intramuscularly, of Glucantime® for 20 days. If necessary, a second or third course can be administered after the initial treatment.

MCL shows a highly variable response to antimonials, and for some authors, there is no cure with this drug. Amphotericin B or pentamidin are better alternatives. In a recent publication, good results were observed in 10 patients with MCL treated with an association of meglumine antimoniate and pentoxifylline (19).

In our experience, pentamidin is the first-line therapy for both LCL and MCL. The recommended dose is 4 mg/kg intramuscularly, every two days in a total of three courses. The same dose is used for MCL, administered 10 times. Once the therapy is completed, the patient is followed with ELISA titles every 6 months.

Amphotericin B is the second or third therapeutic option for LCL. It is a very important drug for difficult to treat cases of MCL. The dose is 1.0 mg/kg intravenously every other day, in a total of 2-3 g. The patient must be hospitalized to be treated with this drug.

Other described systemic treatments are prolonged high-dose of oral ketoconazole, fluconazole, rifampicin and miltefosine.

Several local therapeutic approaches have been reported. The topical application of paromomycin sulfate, an aminoglycoside antibiotic that proved to be effective against leishmanial parasites in vitro, remains controversial. Intralesional application of pentavalent antimony compounds, including sodium stibogluconate and meglumine antimonite have shown response rates between 72% and 100%. A good response of cutaneous leishamaniasis was also described with the use of CO_2 lasers. In a recent trial with 132 patients, this modality was statistically more effective than treatment with Glucantime®. Other surgical approaches include cryotherapy, excision, curettage and eletrodissecation. Experimental approaches, such as photodynamic therapy are also reported; however, further studies are required to prove the efficacy of this method.

REFERENCES

1   Desjeux P. The increased incidence in risk factors for leishmaniasis worldwide. *Trans R Soc Trop Med Hyg* 2001;95:239-43.

2   El-Hassan AM, Zijlstra EE. Leishmaniasis in Sudan. Cutaneous leishmaniasis. *Trans Roy Soc Trop Med Hyg* (Suppl 1) 2001;95:S1/1-S1/17.

3   Boecken GH. New world tegumental leishmaniasis in Brazil: with special reference to the situation of the disease in Manaus, Central Amazon Basin. Thesis. London School of Hygiene and Tropical Medicine, 1996.

4   Oliveira Guerra JA de, Talhari S, Paes MG, Garrido M, Talhari JM. Clinical and diagnostic aspects of American tegumentary leishmaniasis in soldiers simultaneously exposed to the infection in the Amazon region. *Rev Soc Bras Med Trop* 2003;36:587-90.

5   Altamirano-Ensiso AJ, Marzochi MC, Moreira JS, Schubach AO, Marzochi KB. On the origin and spread of cutaneous and mucosal leishmaniasis, based on pre- and post- colombian historical source. *Hist Scienc Saude Manguinhos* 2003;10:852-82.

6   Cruz I, Morales MA, Noguer I, Rodriguez A, Alvar J. Leishmania in discarded syringes from intravenous drug users. *Lancet* 2002;359:1124-5.

7   Silveira FT, Moraes MAP, Shaw JJ, Lainson R. Pathology and pathogenesis of cutaneous leishmaniasis of man in the Amazon Region of Brazil caused by Leishmania (Leishmania) amazonensis. *Acta Parasitol Turcica* 1997;21:97-8.

8   Silveira FT, Lainson R, Corbett CE. Clinical and immunopathological spectrum of American cutaneous leishmaniasis with special reference to the disease in Amazonian Brazil: a review. *Mem Inst Oswaldo Cruz* 2004;99:239-51.

9   Machado P, Kanitakis J, Almeida R, Chalon A, Araujo C, Carvalho EM. Evidence of in situ citotoxicity in American cutaneous leishmaniasis. *Eur J Dermatol* 2002;12:449-51.

10 Scott P, Artis D, Uzonna J, Zaph C. The development of effector and memory T cells in cutaneous leishmaniasis: the implication for vaccine development. *Immunol Rev* 2004;201:318-38.

11 Romero GAS, Farias Guerra MV de, Paes MG, Oliveira Macedo V de. Comparison of cutaneous leishmaniasis due to *Leishmania (Viannia) braziliensis* and *L. (V.) guyansensis* in Brazil: Clinical findings and diagnostic approach. *Clin Infect Dis* 2001;32:1304-12.

12 Puig L, Pradinaud R. Leishmania and HIV co-infection: dermatological manifestations. *Ann Trop Med Parasitol* 2003;97(suppl.):107-14.

13 Turetz ML, Machado PR, KO AI, Alves F, Bittencourt A, Almeidaq RP, Mobashery N, Johnson WD jr, Carvalho EM. Disseminated leishmaniasis: A new and emerging form of leishmaniasis observed in northeastern Brazil. *J Infect Dis* 2002;186:1828-34.

14 Oliveira CI, Fabica A, Oliveira F, Favali CBF, Correa T, Freitas LAR, Nascimento E, Costa JM, Barral A. Clinical utility of polymerase chain reaction-based detection of Leishmania in the diagnosis of american cutaneous leishmaniasis. *Clin Infect Dis* 2003;37:149-53.

15 Davies CR, Llano-Cuentas EA, Campos P, Monge J, Leon E, Canales J. Spraying houses in the Peruvian Andes with lambda-cyhalothrin protects residents against cutaneous leishmaniasis. *Trans Roy Soc Trop Med Hyg* 2000;94:631-6.

16 Reyburn H, Ashford R, Mohsen M, Hewitt S, Rowland M. A randomized controlled trial of insecticide-treated bednets and chaddars or top sheets, and residual spraying of interior rooms for the prevention of cutaneous leishmaniasis in Kabul, Afghanistan. *Trans R Soc Trop Med Hyg* 2000;94:361-6.

17 Blum J, Desjeux P, Schwaqrtz E, Beck B, Hatz C. Treatment of cutaneous leishmaniasis among travellers. *J Antimicrob Chemother* 2004;53:158-66.

18 Minodier P, Noel G, Blanc P, Uters M, Retornaz K, Garnier JM. Traitement des leishmanioses cutanées de l´adulte et de l´enfant. Med Trop 2005;65:487-95.

19 Lessa HA, Machado P, Lima F, Cruz AA, Bacellar O, Guerreiro J, Carvalho EM. Successful treatment of refractory mucosal leishmaniasis with pentoxifylline plus antimony. *Am J Trop Med Hyg* 2001;65:87-9.

15 Leishmaniasis: old world

F. Vega-López

15.1 INTRODUCTION

The term Old World Cutaneous Leishmaniases(OWCL) is given to a group of parasitic diseases caused by protozoan flagellate organisms of the genus *Leishmania* order Kinetoplastida, family Trypanosomatidae. Cutaneous leishmaniasis affects humans as well as a variety of wild and domestic animals that function as a reservoir in the transmission cycle as this is commonly a zoonosis. However, in some instances the affected human can be the source of infection in an anthroponotic cycle, such as observed in Afghanistan and Sudan in cases of localised simple cutaneous infection by *Leishmania tropica* or else cases of post-kala-azar dermal leishmaniasis (PKDL) caused by *L. donovani* in India and Sudan. The parasites are transmitted to humans by the infective bite of the phlebotomine sand fly and particular species of vectors are adapted to transmit particular species of the parasite that subsequently determines the type of clinical disease. The main species of leishmanial parasites causing disease in the old world are: *L. major, L. tropica, L. aethiopica, L. donovani donovani* and *L.d. infantum.*

Each form of clinical leishmaniasis manifests distinct features that make them individually different from the other types within the spectrum. They are unique in etiology transmission, vector, reservoirs, epidemiology, and geographical distribution. These individual features are also relevant to design an effective therapeutic intervention and to establish the expected prognosis. This chapter presents a brief summary of the most important individual features from recently described research on particular *Leishmania* species and this is followed by a practical general discussion on epidemiology, clinical/laboratory diagnosis, treatment and control.

15.2 EPIDEMIOLOGY

15.2.1 L. major

This is the main cause of localised simple cutaneous leishmaniasis in an endemic pattern as found in Iran, North Morocco, Algeria, Middle East, North India, Pakistan, Central Asia and sub-Saharan Africa. This species is also responsible for outbreaks of cutaneous simple leishmaniasis in Iran, Sabzevar county, where surveys in children have found a prevalence of 9% for scars and 6% for active ulcers. This is a zoonotic infection and *Rhombomys opimus* has been found to be the main reservoir host and *P. papatasi* the main vector (1).With regards to virulence factors, it has been described that *L. major* protein disulfide isomerase is particularly expressed in virulent strains and enzymatic inhibitors have resulted in lower virulence and decreased parasitic growth (2). Phosphoglycans also play a role in the persistence of parasites for a long time and are involved in disease expression. In view that *L. major* infections tend to be universally self-healing it has been postulated and found that the infection induces a CD4+ Th1 helper immune response which initially controls and limits infection and subsequently confers permanent immunity to reinfection by the same species.

Professional antigen presenting cells in the host are a main feature of the Th1 protective immune response in leishmaniasis and this role has been demonstrated in experimental systems. Dendritic cells are important to transport *leishmania* parasites and signals of the infection from the skin to local lymph nodes in mice models and this role has been confirmed in both Langerhans and plasmacytoid cells. The acute inflammatory cellular infiltrate also plays a significant role as infected neutrophils secrete chemokines to attract macrophages that ultimately become the host cells for *leishmania* parasites (3).

15.2.2 L. tropica

L. tropica causes localised or disseminated simple cutaneous leishmaniasis in Eastern Mediterranean and sub-Mediterranean regions. This species is widely found in cases from Northern Morocco, Central Asia, Afghanistan, Pakistan, Iraq, Kashmir, and Saudi Arabia. The infection is commonly transmitted through an anthroponotic cycle in urban Asian communities (Kabul, Peshawar). For many years now, it has been recognised that different strains of *L. tropica* have the ability to induce a variable spectrum of clinical disease, i.e. cutaneous, mucosal, visceral or viscerotropic clinical pictures. Most commonly skin lesions are non-ulcerative and non-progressive, however, cases have been reported with an exceptionally virulent and chronic clinical course. There seems to be a specific enzymatic compound that determines the variable spectrum of disease (4). Cysteine proteases from *L. tropica* are virulence factors that are essential for growth and pathogenicity of amastigotes in the mammalian host. Different authors have found mucosal leishmaniasis in children in Saudi Arabia caused by *L. tropica* and in certain regions of the Middle East such as Jordan, particular zymodemes have been described as a cause of simple cutaneous infection. Finally, there is a well recognised clinical picture that seems to result from hypersensitivity to leishmanial antigens and particularly seen in 0.5% to 4% of children with cured localised infection. This small proportion of children and adults with healed *L. tropica* infections develop leishmaniasis *recidivans* also called lupoid leishmaniasis particularly on the face, several years after cure (5).

15.2.3 L. aethiopica

L. aethiopica infection manifests in two different clinical forms, self-healing localised cutaneous and anergic diffuse cutaneous leishmaniasis. Cutaneous leishmaniasis is endemic in Ethiopia, Kenya, Eastern Sudan, and South West Africa, however, this species has also been identified in wild reservoirs in Saudi Arabia (6). The overall prevalence of localised cutaneous infections on the Western side of Ethiopian Rift Valley has been identified in 4% of general population and 8.5% in the age group 0 to 10 years. Approximately 50% of clinical cases suffer active disease for 9 months and 10% for over 3 years and scars are present in up to 35% of residents. A positive leishmanin skin test has been found in 55% of children without signs of disease and *Phlebotomus pedifer* has been identified as the only vector for *L. aethiopica* (7).

In view that this particular species causes localised or diffuse anergic forms of clinical disease, efforts have been directed at the identification of virulence factors or genetic variability within the species. DNA PCR fingerprinting techniques have disclosed ample genetic heterogeneity that correlates with the geographical distribution, however, the polymorphism does not seem to be responsible for the different clinical pictures observed in different hosts and a total of 10 different strains have been described to date.

In vitro evidence shows that promastigotes from patients with localised disease induce Th1 cytokines, whereas those from anergic cases, where antigen specific nonresponsiveness is found, the cytokine pattern reveals a Th0 or Th2 type of response. Ultrastructural studies have revealed that both parasites and host's cells differ widely depending on whether they are from localised or diffuse cutaneous leishmaniasis cases. Cases with diffuse anergic illness are characterized by macrophages with larger parasitophorous vacuoles, higher number of amastigotes per vacuole, larger promastigotes and larger amastigotes. It has been demonstrated that in non-human primate experimental systems the active lesions and subsequent healing of localised infections, are followed by an effective DTH reaction and permanent immunity to challenge by parasites from localised or diffuse cases. Murine models have confirmed that the control of infection involves a successful DTH reaction in both skin and lymphatic tissues.

Finally, research has shown that the IgG antibody response from patients with diffuse cutaneous leishmaniasis recognises antigens of higher molecular mass (~ 90 kDa) than those recognised by cases with localised infections (~ < 25 kDa). Healed localised cutaneous leishmaniasis by *L. aethiopica* may relapse many years after cure following infection by HIV.

15.2.4 L. donovani donovani and L. donovani infantum

The first of these species is responsible for visceral leishmaniasis and relevant to dermatologists in that it causes PKDL in India, Bangladesh, Nepal, and in Africa, particularly Sudan. *L. donovani infantum* can also cause visceral leishmaniasis, however, it commonly determines localised or disseminated cutaneous leishmaniasis in the Western Mediterranean basin including all Southern European countries. *L.d. infantum* has been reported to cause pure lymphadenitis without any skin involvement. A high number of asymptomatic individuals in the general population have been infected, as determined by positive leishmanin skin test in Tunisia (45 to 80% of subjects), as well as in Spain where random serology in Castilla-Leon revealed a 5% of positive seroprevalence, with even higher values of up to 64% in those with HIV infection (8).

The role of symptomatic or asymptomatic dogs as domestic reservoirs in *L.d. infantum* infection has been well recognised and characterized in Mediterranean European and African countries. Serological surveys in Algiers have found 37% positive mostly asymptomatic dogs by IFAT, and a similar picture was described in Greece (9). On the contrary, there is a minimal or absent risk of infection for Northern European dogs taken on holidays to Mediterranean countries.

Most cases of *L.d. infantum* are transmitted by *Phlebotomus perniciosus*, and *P. longicuspis* in this area (10).

Epidemiological and laboratory based research on the variable clinical expression of *L.d. infantum* infections has described a high number of strains within this particular species. Over a period of 10 years for instance, a total of 20 different strains have been recognised by zymodeme analysis in Spain (11), and specific investigations in HIV infected individuals have reported 20 zymodemes in visceral and cutaneous leishmaniasis by the same parasite in 15 years (12).

The above variability has further biological implications as it has been observed that parasites causing infection in immunocompromised individuals have different DNA sequences than those isolated from an immunocompetent host, suggesting that this difference may be responsible for the increased pathogenicity in the immunocompromised.

15.2.5 PKDL

This is a particular type of dermatosis that manifests during or after treatment and commonly following clinical cure of visceral leishmaniasis. The affected lesional, but not the healthy looking skin tissue, contains amastigotes, antigenic products, or *L. donovani* DNA which are useful to make a positive diagnosis. PKDL is highly relevant in the anthroponotic cycle of visceral leishmaniasis infection and is very uncommon in the context of HIV co-infection. In spite of the fact that the immunology of PKDL is not completely understood, a limited body of evidence from research suggests that this dermatosis results from the attack of the immune system to surviving amastigotes in the skin after treatment. It has been found that following treatment of visceral leishmaniasis the peripheral blood mononuclear cells produce IFN-γ and this coincides with the appearance of PKDL. It has also been reported that high concentrations of IL-10 during visceral leishmaniasis infection predicts the development of PKDL, and that CD4+ T helper lymphocytes are decreased in number when compared to CD8+ cells in hypopigmented PKDL skin lesions. Finally, cases with HIV co-infection with visceral leishmaniasis have been reported to develop PKDL following immune recovery from HAART.

There are two main types of PKDL with unique features i.e. the Indian and the African types. The former has been described in India, Bangladesh and Nepal and it is prevalent in hyperendemic areas with visceral leishmaniasis such as Bihar.

This type manifests in approximately 5 to 10% of cases with visceral leishmaniasis and the clinical picture of PKDL follows the visceral disease in 2 or 3 years, however, cases can manifest after 10 years of the treated episode with visceral leishmaniasis. Indian PKDL always requires treatment with antimonials for 4 months or more.

The African type of PKDL has been observed in Sudan, Kenya and East Africa and cases can be caused by *L. donovani donovani* or *L. donovani infantum*. PKDL has been recorded in up to 50% of cases with visceral leishmaniasis in Sudan where *P. orientalis* is the main vector and the onset of the dermatological manifestations takes place at the time or within six months of the visceral episode. PKDL is particularly severe in children and a number of clinical observations have found increased morbidity and mortality in the presence of malnutrition, anaemia below 9 g/dL haemoglobin, high levels of CRP, splenomegaly, diarrhoea, vomiting, or bleeding. PKDL can heal spontaneously within one year and genetic susceptibility to both visceral disease and PKDL has been suspected in Sudan.

15.3 EPIDEMIOLOGY, GEOGRAPHIC DISTRIBUTION, ETIOLOGY AND MODE OF INFECTION IN OLD WORLD CUTANEOUS LEISHMANIASIS

OWCL are distributed in most of the Mediterranean basin (Southern Europe, Asia Minor, Northern Africa), the Middle East, Central Asia, parts of India, China, and a few countries in sub-Saharan Africa. The disease has been found in 62 Old World countries and the World Health Organization has estimated that 500 000 new cases of cutaneous leishmaniasis occur worldwide every year.

The *Leishmania* parasite is a dimorphic protozoan that occurs as a flagellated promastigote with an approximate size of 25 x 3 µm living within the sand fly's intestinal tract. The infective form inside the host's macrophages manifests as a 2-6 µm in size, oval or round amastigote. The *Leishmania* parasites present in the skin of humans or animal reservoirs as amastigotes are taken up with a blood meal by the female Phlebotomine sandfly (Diptera). At least 40 different species of Phlebotomine sand flies relevant in the transmission of leishmaniasis have been described in the Old World. Following ingestion, the protozoan organisms undergo a process of differentiation in the vector's rear- or mid-gut that takes a few days for most species and they finally reach the stage of infective metacyclic promastigote present in the salivary glands of the sandfly. The inoculum with infective promastigotes is transmitted through the bite of female sand flies while taking the next blood meal from the vessels in the superficial dermis of a new host. A variety of factors such as the size of the inoculum, number of bites, and the host's genetic, nutritional and immunological status determine the outcome of overt clinical disease or else elimination of the parasites without any symptomatic manifestation. For those who develop clinical illness within the next few weeks following the infective bite, this may manifest as localised simple cutaneous leishmaniasis, disseminated picture with multiple lesions, anergic forms of diffuse cutaneous leishmanisis, or else PKDL that starts at the time or months following systemic treatment for visceral leishmaniasis.

Apart from humans that are relevant as reservoirs in anthroponotic cases of leishmaniasis there is la large number of wild and domestic hosts in the zoonotic transmission of the disease. The most commonly identified hosts include gerbils, hamsters, mice, rats, foxes, dogs, donkeys, and goats. In particular, dogs represent the most important domestic reservoir for infections by *L. donovani* complex in the Mediterranean basin.

The OWCL affect individuals of all age groups and both genders as well as entire populations in hyperendemic regions in rural and urban areas. Clinical cases can present sporadically or else in outbreaks or true epidemics such as reported in Kabul, Afghanistan, and Sudan. Numerous population surveys have found high infection rates between 5% and > 80% of the general population in Mediterranean, Asian, and African countries, and several studies have described that children in the Middle East, central Asia, and Sudan have a higher risk to infection and overt cutaneous disease than the general population.

The most used epidemiological tools for surveys are the presence of scar, active skin infection rates, serology, leishmanin skin test, and more recently DNA molecular testing in blood specimens. The incidence and prevalence rates of different types of leishmaniases do not remain constant through time as several factors such as temperature, altitude, rain precipitation, season, sand fly activity, reservoirs, and population movements modify the frequency of infection and ultimately of clinical disease. Apart from the millions of indigenous population at risk, particular groups of individuals become exposed to infective bites when travelling to endemic regions. Cutaneous leishmaniases from both the Old and New Worlds have been reported as an emerging infection for travellers, military personnel, missionaries, visitors, and refugees who may develop the condition upon return to non-endemic regions of the world (13). In the author's experience at the specialised 'Skin Infections and Tropical Dermatology Clinic' (Hospital for Tropical Diseases, London, UK) patients present sporadically and also following mini-outbreaks in dozens of military personnel deployed in endemic regions for *L. tropica* and *L. major*. Risk factors for the traveller

Figure 15.1 Simple old world cutaneous leishmaniasis on the wrist

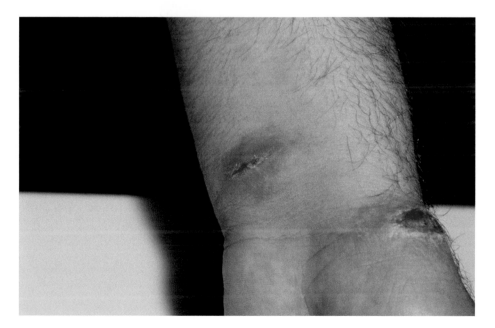

include sleeping outdoors, without a protective net or insect repellents at the time of sand fly activity.

15.4 CLINICAL PICTURE

15.4.1 Localised cutaneous simple leishmaniasis

All of Old World *Leishmania* species can cause this clinical form of disease. On clinical grounds the typical cutaneous elementary lesion in localised leishmaniasis is an ulcer surrounded by an erythemato-violaceous nodular border that fails to heal in weeks or a few months (figure 15.1).

Figure 15.2   Other forms with lymphangitic involvement

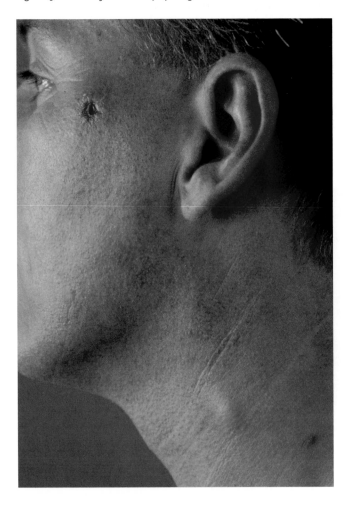

The morphological spectrum however is variable and clinical leishmaniasis may manifest in papular, plaque, nodular, crusted, and pure lymphangitic forms amongst other (figure 15.2).

The clinical symptoms manifest on average between 4 to 12 weeks following the infective sandfly bite and different species induce a variable range of pathogenic potential and timing for events of clinical disease. For instance, *L. major* causes a particular type of rural, zoonotic, wet ulcer that heals spontaneously in 6 to 8 months, whereas lesions caused by *L. tropica* are often described as a dry urban anthroponotic type of disease that can take more than a year to heal and often only after treatment. Nodular, papular, or ulcerated forms caused by *L. aethiopica* can take longer to heal and parasites can be identified in clinical lesions for up to 5 years. The typical sore in simple cutaneous leishmaniasis is circular or oval in shape and measures between 1 and 5 cm in size. Spontaneous healing in simple leishmaniasis results in a flat or atrophic scar with mild erythema that resolves over several months. The healing process may result in milia cyst formation in cases treated by oral purine analogues, intralesional antimonials or in those with spontaneous cure.

The lesions in simple leishmaniasis are predominantly found on exposed regions of skin and on areas with relatively thin skin covering bone prominences such as forehead, mastoidal region, zygoma, chin, wrist, hand dorsum, or malleolar regions. The lesions tend to be asymptomatic, however, pain is common in cases with superimposed bacterial infection, cellulitis, or following recurrent mechanical trauma (figure 15.3).

Figure 15.3   Disseminated leishmaniasis with cellulitis

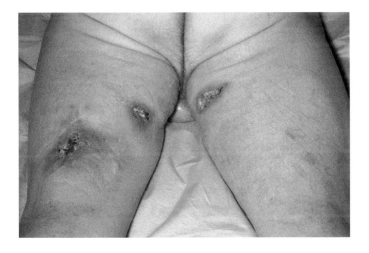

15.4.2 Disseminated and complex cutaneous leishmaniasis

This type is commonly caused by *L. tropica, L. aethiopica, L. donovani infantum* and less commonly by *L. major* infections. The clinical picture and presentation pattern is similar to the localised forms except that several lesions are found on the particular anatomical region and tend to have a prominent lymphangitic component with local and regional lymph node enlargement. An initial single lesion located on an acral part of a limb may disseminate proximally through lymphatics and the timing for new, more recent ulcers becomes obvious on taking the clinical history. Ulcers, crateriform sores, or other type of skin lesion that manifest in different anatomical regions and at about the same time suggest on the other hand, multiple infective bites. Disseminated and complex forms tend to manifest with larger lesions, heavier parasitic load, and longer duration than those found in simple localised disease (figure 15.4). This form of leishmaniasis requires treatment.

15.4.3 Lupoid or recidivans leishmaniasis

This is a chronic form of clinical disease where parasite and DNA-based investigations are negative. The condition is seen in healed lesions by *L. tropica* infection and lasts for several years. It seems that a hypersensitivity reaction to leishmanial antigens results in a papular or nodular eruption several months or a few years after the original sore of simple or complex leishmaniasis. The lupoid lesions commonly appear on the periphery of the scar tissue and tend to progress slowly. The small papules or nodules require treatment with intralesional antimonials, surgical excision, thermosurgery and/or oral allopurinol.

Figure 15.4 Disseminated leishmaniasis

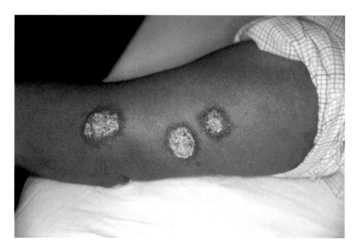

15.4.4 Diffuse cutaneous anergic leishmaniasis

This type of chronic clinical disease caused by *L. aethiopica* adopts a relapsing pattern following treatment. A single original lesion disseminates locally at first and subsequently to different anatomical sites and typically presents with heavy parasitic load and anergy with a lack of DTH response on leishmanin intradermal test. The *Leishmania* parasites can persist for long periods of time after partial therapeutic response and become responsible for severe disease upon reactivation.

15.4.5 PKDL

PKDL disease appears late after clinical cure of Visceral Leishmaniasis (VL). The morphological clinical features include hypopigmented patches or plaques, maculo-papular rash, erythematous eruptions, nodules, lichenoid eruptions, verrucous plaques, few or numerous, disseminated and affecting trunk and limbs. The skin lesions can start around the mouth and then disseminate to the trunk and limbs and on the face they can also cause ocular involvement with blepharitis, conjunctivitis and uveitis. Cases have been described with generalised lymphadenopathy and the skin lesions can occur more frequently and be worse in sun exposed areas, however, involvement of mucosal areas in nasopharynx, oral, genital, ano-rectal and laryngeal vocal chords has been described. Most of the patients with the African type heal spontaneously within one year, whereas the disease requires treatment in all Indian type cases. In general, the disease is more severe in children. The clinical features and the temporal relationship between the VL and PKDL signs together with the demonstration of parasites in lesional skin are the pillars for a positive diagnosis.

15.5 DIFFERENTIAL CLINICAL DIAGNOSIS

Simple and complex leishmaniases may reveal identical or very similar clinical features to a number of other cutaneous infectious and non-infectious disorders. Some of the commonest differentials include *M. marinum* and other tuberculous and NTM infections, sporotrichosis, leprosy, pyogenic infections, ecthyma, mycetoma, cutaneous diphtheria, anthrax, sarcomata, lymphoma, BCC, SCC, malignant melanoma, keratoacanthoma, actinic reticuloid, poikiloderma, and papular eruptions. Lupoid leishmaniasis can be identical to lupus vulgaris or sarcoidosis, and diffuse anergic leishmaniasis to lepromatous leprosy. PKDL has to be differentiated from a large list of skin diseases including leprosy, lymphoma, sarcomata, sarcoidosis, vitiligo, pinta, pellagra, miliaria rubra, syphilis, and onchocerciasis amongst other conditions.

15.6 DIAGNOSTIC PROCEDURES

A positive diagnosis of leishmaniasis on clinical grounds is quite simple in endemic regions of the world where the general population and the health personnel are familiarised with the clinical course and symptoms. The returning traveller to non-endemic regions, however, presents a challenge due to a lack of training and knowledge on this condition in extra-leishmanial latitudes. The gold standard for diagnosis is the presence of parasites in lesional skin and there are a number of investigations to demonstrate this, however, the diagnosis can be supported by several or in some cases by one of the criteria listed below (14). Two of the most important factors for a positive diagnosis are firstly, the correct sampling of lesional skin carried out by an experienced clinician and secondly, to be aware that a diagnosis of leishmaniasis can be firmly established in the absence of parasites.

- History of exposure in endemic region in previous weeks or months.
- History of sand fly bites in the previous weeks or months.
- History of high risk activities such as jungle/desert trekking or sleeping outdoors.
- Presence of non-healing, nodular, violaceous ulcer for 4 to 6 weeks or much longer.
- Presence of a non-healing skin lesion and local/regional lymphatic tissue involvement in the context of relevant history of exposure in an endemic area.
- Presence of amastigotes in Giemsa-stained smears from lesional skin.
- Demonstration of intracellular amastigotes in the dermis of HE skin specimens.
- Presence of leishmanial granulomata in the dermis of HE skin specimens.
- Growth of promastigotes from lesional skin in NNN culture medium.
- Demonstration of leishmanial DNA by PCR in lesional skin.

In view of the fact that a positive parasitological or molecular diagnosis is not always available or possible, the author has found that a combination of investigations can lead to a definite diagnosis of leishmaniasis. In order to achieve a fast, specific, sensitive, and species-specific diagnosis all cases with clinical cutaneous leishmaniasis have to be subjected to at least 4 different laboratory tests:

- Giemsa-stained slit skin smear, ulcer scrapings, or biopsy imprint smear.
- Parasitological culture in Novy-MacNeal-Nicolle medium.
- Histopathological investigation on H&E slides.
- Molecular diagnosis to identify species-specific DNA by the PCR.

Additional serological or intradermal leishmanin (Montenegro reaction) testing can be required for patients with PKDL, *L. donovani* infections, the immunocompromised host, and as a tool for seroepidemiological surveys.

In the author's experience and based on published literature the identification of amastigotes by Giemsa-stained smears has a low sensitivity (50-70%) whereas the presence of granuloma in H&E skin biopsy specimens scores higher at around 70% (without amastigotes) to 100% (presence of amastigotes). The histological investigation has the advantage of offering a specific diagnosis as other granulomatous conditions, infectious and non-infectious, can be readily identified or ruled out. On the other hand, the slit skin smears are easy to use in field conditions where direct microscopy is available for an instant diagnosis. In spite of the fact that both methods are widely available in most endemic regions of the Old World, they are not conclusive with regards the identification of leishmanial species or sub-species. The parasitological culture requires basic laboratory technology and once the promastigotes develop in a few days, it has the advantage to allow for the identification of particular species by PCR-based methods or else by zymodeme analysis in a reference laboratory. The culture of particular *Leishmania* species can be unsatisfactory and this is due to a variety of reasons including bacterial and fungal contaminants, chronicity of specimen, sampling specimen with a low parasitic burden, all of which may result in a decreased diagnostic sensitivity.

Several PCR methods to identify leishmanial DNA have been available for over a decade and they have been adapted for clinical laboratory and field-based diagnosis. Most of the currently used PCR methods however, use leishmanial minicircle DNA. Specimens of any kind from lesional skin can be successfully used including frozen or paraffin-embedded skin, cotton swab exudate, fresh or archival Giemsa smears, material from fine needle aspiration, and lesional skin or exudates in lysis buffer or ethanol. Most authors have reported a PCR overall sensitivity between 90-100% of cases with the advantage of the identification of species and sub-species if appropriate primers are available. A few surveys however, have found very low sensitivity in chronic cases.

Serological tests are mainly used to diagnose visceral leishmaniasis and have been useful in PKDL. A number of *L.d. infantum* recombinant antigens have been characterized for diagnosis and a direct agglutination test (DAT) can be useful in the diagnosis of cutaneous leishmaniasis by *L. aethiopica* with sensitivity of 90-92% specificity.

15.7 TREATMENT

Overall most cases of simple cutaneous leishmaniasis caused by any of the Old World species, can be cured by 6 to 10 weekly intralesional injections of sodium stibogluconate (inject 0.5 to 1.5 ml of 100 mg/ml sodium stibogluconate solution, once weekly). In cases where intradermal injections are not feasible or acceptable, a number of orally administered purine analogues (allopurinol 10 to 20 mg/kg/day/8 to 10 weeks) or antifungals can result in clinical cure (itraconazole 100 to 200 mg/day; terbinafine 250 mg/day; fluconazole 150 mg/day; all for 8 to 10 weeks or until 2 weeks after clinical cure). A considerable number of cases of simple cutaneous leishmaniasis by *L. major* or *L. tropica* affecting individuals in endemic regions heal spontaneously and are never treated. The burden of poverty, poor education, and the lack of diagnostic or therapeutic facilities determine the above. Other successful therapeutic approaches in simple small lesions include cryotherapy, surgical excision, thermosurgery, and topical 15% paromomycin in paraffin with aminoglucoside antibiotics or urea.

Infections with complex lesions caused by any of the Old World species require systemic treatment or else a combination of drugs. Intravenous pentavalent antimonial (Pentostam®) is the drug of choice and is administered by IV daily infusion at 20 mg/kg/21 to 28 days for complex lesions. Cases with African PKDL require 2 months and those of Indian PKDL several months. In cases of diffuse cutaneous leishmaniasis by *L. aethiopica* pentamidine at 4 mg/kg/week for as long as necessary is first therapeutic choice. *L. aethiopica* infections in Kenya have been treated by Pentostam® at 18-20 mg/kg twice daily for 30 days with a successful therapeutic outcome and no relapse.

Pentavalent antimonials have a rapid absorption and excretion and disrupt the synthesis of macromolecules in parasite cells. Amastigotes have a greater sensitivity to antimonials than promastigotes and sodium stibogluconate cumulates in the macrophage secondary lysosomes following leishmanial infection. Adverse effects include shivers, skin rash, fever, myalgia, arthralgia, pancreatitis, hepatitis and cardiotoxicity. Close monitoring, blood investigations, ECG, and experience are essential when administering these compounds.

Allopurinol has an antiprotozoal activity as leishmanial enzymes display high affinity for this compound that inhibits and disrupts the protein synthesis. It has been successfully used in combination with intralesional or intravenous antimonials to treat both cutaneous and visceral leishmaniasis. In the author's experience, therapeutic failures to IV Pentostam® (*L. tropica*, *L. Viannia braziliensis*, and *L. mexicana* complex infections) have responded to a combined regime with intralesional weekly Pentostam® injections and oral allopurinol for 8 to 12 weeks. This regime has also been successful to treat cases with chronic lupoid leishmaniasis by *L. tropica*.

Triazole and allylamine antifungals disrupt the ergosterol synthesis and azoles have been found to be active against several species of leishmania promastigotes and to a lesser extent versus amastigotes. The disruption of the membrane and metabolic function has been observed against *L. donovani*, *L. braziliensis* and *L. amazonensis*. Ketoconazole exhibits good effect against *L. mexicana*, and most azoles are efficacious in *L. major* infections.

Amphotericin B and liposomal amphotericin are effective in VL and PKDL. This is a polyene antibiotic that disrupts the plasma membrane of the parasite cell. It has been used as a second choice in cases resistant to antimonials and particularly for intractable cases of cutaneous and mucocutaneous leishmaniasis or those with HIV co-infection. Amphotericin B is used at a dose of 1 mg/kg body weight/day. On the other hand the liposomal preparation results in decreased toxicity and higher plasma concentrations and ambisome at a dose of 2 mg/kg body weight in days 1 to 4 and day 10 has resulted in 90% cure in cases of VL.

15.8 PREVENTION

Prevention and control measures are directed at several levels: host, vectors, reservoirs and environment. Common initiatives include the use of one or several of the following strategies: protective clothing, insecticide-treated nets, avoidance of bites, protection during sleep, control of rubbish, control reservoirs, early diagnosis, residual spraying of animal shelters and households, impregnated dog collars. Resistance to DDT insecticide by *Phlebotomus papatasi* and *P. argentipes* has been reported in India. Imidacloprid/permethrin combination of repellent/insecticide for dogs is highly effective.

REFERENCES

1   Yaghoobi-Ershadi MR, Akhavan AA, Zahraei-Ramazani AV, Abai MR, Ebrahimi B, Jafari R. Epidemiological study in a new focus of cutaneous leishmaniasis in the Islamic Republic of Iran. *East Mediterr Health J* 2003;9:816-26.

2   Ben Achour Y, Chenik M, Louzir H, Dellagi K. Identification of a disulfide isomerase protein of *Leishmania major* as a putative virulence factor. *Infect Immunity* 2002;70:3576-85.

3   Zandbergen G van, Klinger M, Mueller A, Dannenberg S, Gebert A, Solbach W, Laskay T. Cutting edge: neutrophil granulocyte serves as a vector for Leishmania entry into macrophages. *J Immunol* 2004;173:6521-5.

4   Lira R, Mendez S, Carrera L, Jaffe C, Neva F, Sacks D. *Leishmania tropica*: the identification and purification of metacyclic promastigotes and use in establishing mouse and hamster models of cutaneous and visceral disease. *Experim Parasitol* 1998;89:331-42.

5   Bowling JC and Vega-López F. Lupoid leishmaniasis 2003. *Clin Exp Dermatol* 28:683-84.

6   Morsy TA, al Dakhil MA, el Bahrawy AF. Characterisation of *Leishmania aethiopica* from rock hyrax, Procavia capensis trapped in Najran, Saudi Arabia. *J Egypt Soc Parasitol* 1997;27:349-53.

7   Mengistu G, Laskay T, Gemetchu T, Humber D, Ersamo M, Evans D, Teferedegn H, Phelouzat MA, Frommel D. Cutaneous leishmaniasis in south-western Ethiopia: Ocholo revisited. *Trans Roy Soc Trop Med Hyg* 1992;86:149-53.

8   Garrote JI, Gutierrez MP, Izquierdo RL, Duenas MA, Zarzosa P, Cañabate C, Bali ME, Almaraz A, Bratos MA, Berbel C, Domingo AO. Seroepidemiologic study of *Leishmania infantum* infection in Castilla-Leon, Spain. *Am J Trop Med Hyg* 2004;71:403-6.

9   Papadopoulou C, Kostuola A, Dimitriou D, Panagiou A. Human and canine leishmaniasis in asymptomatic and symptomatic population in Northwestern Greece. *J Infect* 2005;50:53-60.

10 Harrat Z, Belkaid M. Leishmaniasis in Algiers: epidemiologic data. *Bull Soc Pathol Exot* 2003; 96:212-4.

11 Martin-Sanchez J, Gramiccia M, Di Muccio T, Ludovisi A, Morilla-Marquez F. Isoenzymatic polymorphism of *Leishmania infantum* in southern Spain. *Transact Roy Soc Trop Med Hyg* 2004;98:228-32.

12 Pratlong F, Dereure J, Deniau M, Marty P, Dedet JP. Enzymatic polymorphism during Leishmania/HIV co-infection: a study of 381 leishmania strains received between 1986 and 2000 at the international cryobank in Montpellier, France. *Ann Trop Med Parasitol* 2003;97 (Suppl 1):47-56.

13 Jones J, Bowling J, Watson J, Vega-López F, White J, Higgins E. Old World cutaneous leishmaniasis in children: a case series. *Arch Dis Child* 2005;90:530-1.

14 Vega-López F. Diagnosis of cutaneous leishmaniasis. *Curr Opin Infect Dis* 2003;16:97-101.

15 Vega-López F, Hay R. Parasitic Worms and Protozoa. In: Burns T, Breathnach S, Cox N, Griffiths C (ed.). Rook's Textbook of Dermatology - London (UK): Blackwell Publishing, 2004: 32.1-32.48.

16 Onchocerciasis / Filariasis

M.E. Murdoch

16.1 GENERAL

16.1.1 Introduction

Filariae (nematodes or roundworms) are responsible for devastating problems in man, including blindness, itchy unsightly rashes and elephantiasis with over 150 million infected people in tropical and sub-tropical regions. There are three main diseases: lymphatic filariasis, is usually caused by *Wuchereria bancrofti,* (in certain areas of the world it is caused by *Brugia malayi* and *B. timori*), onchocerciasis is caused by *O. volvulus* and loiasis by *Loa loa.* Most recent WHO estimates indicate that there are 120 million infected people with lymphatic filariasis, 25 million with *Loa loa* and 17.7 million with onchocerciasis. The other filarial species than can infect man are *Mansonella streptocerca, M. perstans,* and *M. ozzardi.* Skin manifestations are a prominent feature in returned travellers with filarial infection.

16.1.2 Epidemiology

Geographical distribution

Lymphatic filariasis occurs in at least 80 tropical countries in Africa, Asia, South America and the Pacific. *B. timori* is found in small foci in Indonesia and *B. malayi* in Southeast Asia and the Far East. Onchocerciasis is endemic in 28 countries in sub-Saharan Africa and smaller foci also exist in Central and Southern America (Mexico, Guatemala, Ecuador, Colombia, Venezuela and Brazil) and the Yemen (figure 16.1). Loiasis is limited to Central and West Africa (mostly Cameroon, Democratic Republic of Congo, Angola, Gabon, Central African Republic, Nigeria, Chad and Sudan). Infection with *M. streptocerca* occurs in West and Central Africa. *M. perstans* is endemic in much of tropical Africa and South America and parts of the Caribbean. *M. ozzardi* infection occurs only in the American continent in the West Indies, Central America and South America (northern Argentina, Brazil, Colombia, Ecuador, and Peru). Filarial infections are relatively rare in travellers. Figure 16.2 shows the total

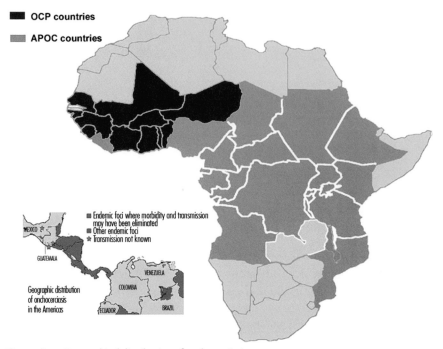

Figure 16.1   Geographical distribution of onchocerciasis

Figure 16.2   Total laboratory reports of filariasis by genus, England, Wales and Northern Ireland: 1990-2004

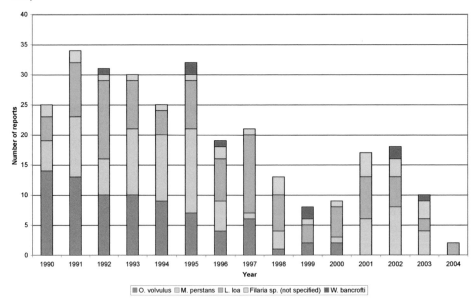

number of laboratory reports of filariasis by genus between 1990 and 2004 for England, Wales and Northern Ireland. National surveillance of laboratory-confirmed infections are reported via LabBase to the Communicable Disease Surveillance Centre (CDSC), Colindale, London but as this is a voluntary system the reports are likely to under-estimate the true burden of travel-associated filarial infection. The main organisms responsible for filarial infection in England, Wales and Northern Ireland are *O. volvulus, L. loa* and *M. perstans*. Further information about which endemic countries were visited is rather limited as 'recent travel history' and 'resort country' are not mandatory core surveillance data fields and hence are often poorly completed. Another difficulty is the inability to distinguish UK travellers from new entrants/migrants. Of the 294 reports between 1990 and 2004, only 80 (27%) specified 'yes' in the field for recent travel abroad but of those, 70 specified recent travel to Africa, the majority to West Africa, especially Cameroon and Nigeria.

16.1.3 Mode of infection

Infective larvae are deposited into the skin by infected arthropod vectors during a blood meal. The larvae then migrate either to the lymphatics (in lymphatic filariasis) or subcutaneous tissues of the human host's body where they develop into adults which can live for several years. In lymphatic filariasis, the adult worms live in lymphatic vessels and lymph nodes; in onchocerciasis the adults are coiled up within fibrous subcutaneous nodules; in loiasis the adult worms reside in subcutaneous tissue where they migrate actively; adult worms of *M. streptocerca* are found in the dermis and subcutaneous tissue and *M. ozzardi* apparently in subcutaneous tissue and *M. perstans* in body cavities and surrounding tissues. After mating, the adult female worms produce microfilariae which circulate in the blood, except for those of *volvulus* and *M. streptocerca* which concentrate in the skin. The microfilariae of *O. volvulus* also preferentially invade the eye. When the biting insect next collects a blood meal it co-incidentally ingests microfilariae which then undergo further development within the insect into infective larvae. During a subsequent blood meal, the larvae infect the vertebrate host and develop into adults, a slow process which in the case of *Onchocerca* may take up to 18 months. Adult worms of the agents of lymphatic filariasis live for 4-6 years whereas adults of *O. volvulus* live for 10-14 years. The relevant vectors are mosquitoes (*Anopheles, Culex, Aedes* and *Mansonia*) for infections of lymphatic filariasis; *Simulium* blackflies for *O. volvulus*; *Chrysops* tabanid deerflies for *Loa loa*; midges *(Culicoides)* for *M. perstans* and *M. streptocerca* and both midges and blackflies for *M. ozzardi*.

16.1.4 Clinical picture

Expatriate syndrome

It has become increasingly recognised that individuals who have not grown up in endemic areas but visit such regions and acquire a filarial infection may develop prominent symptoms and signs of inflammation rather than the chronic clinical signs typically found in long-term residents. Thus expatriates with lymphatic filariasis develop lymphangitis, lymphadenitis, genital pain (from inflamed lymphatics), urticaria and peripheral eosinophilia. Individuals with onchocerciasis may present with itchy, slightly urticated papules and /or edema of the skin. In loiasis, Calabar swellings, urticaria and occasionally asthma have been documented. The reason for these different clinical manifestations appears to be different host responses to filarial antigens between those with long-standing (including pre-natal) exposure and those who are exposed for the first time. Immigrants to developed countries from endemic areas may present with more typical signs of chronic infection.

16.2 ONCHOCERCIASIS

16.2.1 Clinical picture

Cutaneous signs

The first indication of infection is usually pruritus. Other early manifestations include a papular rash, transient urticaria, arthralgia and fever.

The likeliest scenario facing a doctor in a developed country is that of a patient who has visited an endemic area for a relatively short time and now returned. In this setting a detailed travel history over the previous 1-3 years is essential, as the patient may not have realised the significance of foreign travel which had happened some time before the onset of his/her symptoms. This long time-interval between the visit to an endemic region and the onset of symptoms is due the time required for infective larvae to develop into adult worms. After mating the adult female produces microfilariae which gradually accumulate in number and then start to cause symptoms. Latency periods ranging from 7-18 months have been documented (1,2). Persons who have not grown up in, but have spent many years in endemic areas may present with symptoms within shorter times of leaving the endemic area.

Returned visitors of endemic areas usually present with pruritus and/or an itchy papular rash. The papules are small and often concentrated over one area of the body such as a leg, arm, shoulder or waist (3). Often there is accompanying non-pitting lymphatic-type edema of the limb (1) and swelling can also occur independently in the absence of any rash (4). Sometimes the signs are rather subtle and small itchy pink, slightly urticated papules may be all there is to see (2) (figure 16.3). The clinical findings most closely resemble acute papular dermatitis (APOD) which has been documented in children and young adults who are long-term residents of endemic areas.

Life-long residents in endemic areas may develop a variety of skin lesions which can occur singly or in combination. If such individuals migrate to a developed country then they may also present to a doctor there. The various forms of onchocercal skin disease have been classified into acute papular onchodermatitis (APOD), chronic papular onchodermatitis (CPOD), lichenified onchodermatitis (LOD), atrophy and depigmentation (5).

Acute papular onchodermatitis (APOD)

APOD is common in children and young adults and consists of small itchy monomorphic papules which are usually widely scattered over the upper trunk and arms.

Figure 16.3   A, B Subtle urticated papular rash in a young female returned visitor who presented 14 months after leaving Cameroon (inset – close up of urticated papules)

A

B

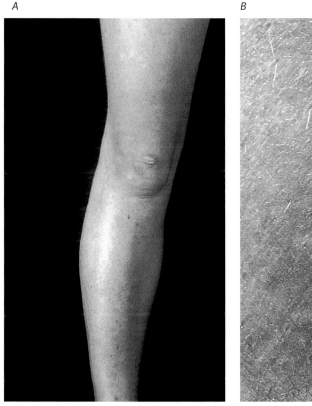
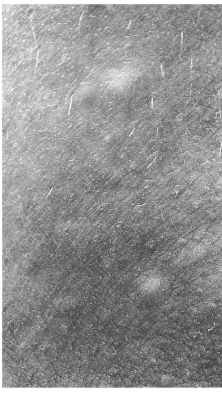

In more severe cases small pustules are seen with or without accompanying edema of the skin causing a peau d'orange appearance.

Chronic papular onchodermatitis (CPOD)

CPOD occurs in children and adults and comprises itchy papules which are larger than those of APOD and more variable in size. They are distributed over the trunk and limbs and are often concentrated around the pelvic girdle. Post-inflammation hyperpigmentation is often present with excoriation (figure 16.4).

Lichenified onchodermatitis (LOD)

LOD is typically found in adolescent boys. It is a localised change usually confined to one limb, particularly the leg. Extremely itchy hyperpigmented papules, nodules and plaques eventually progress into confluent lichenified areas. There is associated swelling of the limb and soft enlargement of the draining lymph nodes.

Atrophy

In order to avoid confusion with normal ageing of the skin, the term onchocercal atrophy is reserved for adults who are less than 50 years old and in whom the skin therefore appears to be prematurely aged. The skin is thin and excessively wrinkled.

Figure 16.4   Chronic papular onchodermatitis in a Nigerian resident of an endemic area

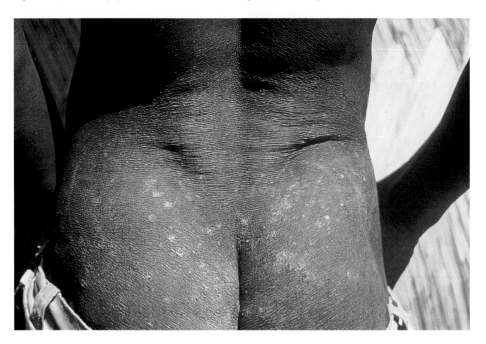

Atrophy is predominantly found around the pelvic girdle and upper thighs. Hanging groin is the specific finding of loose redundant folds of skin in the groin. Atrophy of the skin is not characteristically itchy.

Depigmentation
Patchy depigmentation with 'spots' of normally pigmented skin centred around hair follicles typically occurs over both shins and less frequently in the groins and on genital skin. It is common in older residents of endemic areas and is not itchy.

Onchocercal nodules (onchocercomata)
Residents of endemic areas often have essentially asymptomatic smooth firm subcutaneous nodules ranging from pea-size to several centimetres in diameter. In Africa nodules can be readily palpated over bony prominences such as the iliac crest whereas in Central and South America nodules are more common on the scalp. The nodules consist of coiled adult worms surrounded by a fibrous capsule.

In a multi-country prevalence survey of endemic villages in Africa (6) onchocercal skin disease affected 28% of the population aged 5 years or above. The commonest type was CPOD (13%), followed by depigmentation (10%) and acute papular onchodermatitis (7%). A survey of 83 immigrants in Israel from the Kuwara highland of Northwest Ethiopia, which has a high prevalence of onchocerciasis, revealed that the commonest skin finding was CPOD in more than 46 patients (55%) followed by depigmentation and atrophy (16% and 14% respectively) (7). Skin snips were positive in 40 patients (48%).

Ocular signs
Ocular signs are relatively rare in patients with imported onchocerciasis but it is essential to refer the patient for formal ophthalmological assessment. The easiest way to visualise microfilariae is to ask the patient to adopt a head-down position for 2 min and then examine them on a slit-lamp. Tiny microfilariae may be seen wriggling in the anterior chamber. Live microfilariae in the cornea are more difficult to see as they are transparent. Dead microfilariae in the cornea, however, may be seen as opaque straightened-out microfilariae surrounded by inflammatory infiltrate. These 'fluffy' lesions of punctate keratitis resolve spontaneously. Long-term residents in endemic areas may develop the potentially blinding complications of sclerosing keratitis, iridocyclitis, choroido-retinitis, choroido-retinal atrophy, optic neuritis and optic atrophy. In the study of Ethiopian immigrants in Israel (7), 65 patients underwent a thorough eye examination. Of these 65 patients, 45 patients (69%) had ocular complaints. Corneal abnormalities were detected in 55 of the 130 eyes (42%), active anterior segment inflammation and live microfilariae in 4 eyes (3%) and lens changes in 16 eyes (12%).

Eleven eyes (8%) showed retinal or choroidal changes. Eye manifestations were therefore prevalent among this group of immigrants.

Burden of disease in endemic countries

The socio-economic effects of onchocerciasis are most acute in Africa. The most serious complication is blindness with 270 000 blind and 500 000 people with significant visual loss due to onchocerciasis globally. In endemic areas in Africa, 42% of the adult population have been found to complain of pruritus (6). By extrapolation, an estimated 6 million people in Africa are thought to have troublesome pruritus secondary to onchocerciasis (8). The pruritus is severe, causing insomnia and general debilitation. In endemic regions onchocercal skin disease may have detrimental psycho-social effects (9) and can reduce the marriage prospects of adolescent girls.

16.2.2 Diagnostic procedures

Skin snips

This is the current standard test but it may be negative in pre-patent or light infections as in returned travellers. A small bloodless tent of skin is raised with a needle and the apex shaved off with a scapel. A corneoscleral punch may also be used. The skin snip is placed in saline in the well of a microtitre plate and after 30 min to 24 hours, with the aid of a dissecting microscope, microfilariae may be seen to have migrated out of the tissue. The result may be expressed as just positive or negative or quantified as the number of microfilariae per skin snip. For research purposes skin snips may be weighed and the result expressed as the number of microfilariae per mg of skin. At least one snip is taken from each iliac crest and the sensitivity of the test is increased by taking additional snips from the scapular region and calf.

Other parasitological methods of diagnosis

1   Detection of intra-ocular microfilariae using a slit-lamp, see above.
2   Demonstration of adult worms by histological examination of excised nodules. This is not a routine procedure.
3   Demonstration of microfilariae by histological examination of skin biopsy. Again this is not a routine diagnostic procedure, but if a skin biopsy has been taken, microfilariae may be seen in the upper dermis on routine H & E staining. *O. volvulus* microfilariae have the following distinguishing features: *i)* a cephalic space (7-13 µm) followed by closely approximated anterior nuclei *ii)* a caudal space (9-15 µm) preceded by elongated terminal nuclei and *iii)* a tail with a finely tapered point.

Mazzotti test

If the skin snips are negative, but onchocerciasis is still suspected, the next step is to give a single oral dose of 50 µg of diethylcarbamazine (DEC) and observe the patient carefully. Infected persons may develop intense pruritus 20-90 minutes later. An acute papular rash with edema may develop or an existing rash may be exacerbated. Fever, cough and musculoskeletal symptoms may also occur. Symptoms and signs reach a peak within about 24 hours and gradually subside over the next 48-72 hours. If necessary antihistamines, aspirin and other analgesics may be given for symptomatic relief and occasionally steroids are required for severe symptoms. The Mazzotti test is contraindicated in patients who are heavily infected (who will have positive skin snips) as more severe reactions can occur with pulmonary edema and collapse. The Mazzotti test is also contraindicated in patients with optic nerve disease as it may trigger deterioration in vision.

DEC patch test

This 'Mazzotti' patch test assesses the local reaction of 10% DEC in Nivea® cream or Nivea® milk applied to the skin. It is more sensitive than skin snipping but its use is still being evaluated.

Full blood count

A peripheral eosinophilia may be present.

Future diagnostic methods

Serodiagnosis

A specific serological test for onchocerciasis is not available for routine use yet. A filaria ELISA may be performed but it does not differentiate between the various filarial infections. Specific serological diagnosis for onchocerciasis is an area of current research and it is hoped that a specific diagnostic tool will soon become available using a cocktail of recombinant antigens.

PCR diagnosis

PCR-based assays are only available as research tools at present. PCR is more sensitive than skin-snipping in lightly infected individuals. PCR-based assays to detect the repetitive DNA sequence known as O-150 (found only in *O. volvulus*) has 100% species specificity and 100% sensitivity. PCR has also been shown to detect parasite DNA in skin scrapings.

16.2.3 Treatment

Ivermectin

Lightly infected expatriates with onchocerciasis should be treated with a single dose of 150-200 µg/kg ivermectin with observation in hospital for 72 hours, followed by 2 subsequent doses at monthly intervals (10). In contrast to mass treatment programmes in Africa where reactions are rare, 17/33 (55%) of this series of patients in London had reactions, so it is advisable that the first dose of ivermectin is given in hospital. If there is recurrence of itching, a typical papular rash or eosinophilia, further treatment with ivermectin should be considered at 6-12 monthly intervals. Ivermectin kills microfilariae and has some effect on late stages of embryogenesis of the worms, but as it does not kill the adult worms (which can live for 10-12 years), levels of microfliarae can reaccumulate over many months and treatment has to be repeated.

A large double-blinded multi-country trial in endemic regions in Africa has confirmed the efficacy of ivermectin over placebo in improving pruritus and reduction in prevalence of APOD, CPOD and LOD (11). Ivermectin in this setting was equally effective whether given at 3-monthly, 6-monthly or annual intervals.

Doxycycline

Recently, *Wolbachia* symbiotic endobacteria have been identified as essential for filarial worms' fertility and these offer new targets for therapy.

Additional treatment with doxycycline to sterilise worms thus enhances ivermectin-induced suppression of microfilaridermia. A combination of doxycycline 100 mg/day for 6 weeks plus ivermectin is now advisable for individuals with imported onchocerciasis (12).

Future Treatments

A macrofilaricide which can kill adult worms is desirable so that a single course of treatment could be potentially curative.

16.2.4 Prevention

Prevention of Simulium fly bites

Visitors to endemic areas can limit their exposure to fly bites by keeping away from rivers and banks which are known breeding sites. Protective clothing such as long-sleeved shirts and long trousers and an insect-repellent are advisable especially in the early morning and late evening which are peak biting times.

Control Programmes

The global control of onchocerciasis is dependent upon strategies to reduce the level of disease in endemic areas until it is no longer a significant public health problem.

The WHO Onchocerciasis Control Programme (OCP) 1974-2002

This major programme covering 11 West African countries has successfully eliminated the vector blackfly by aerial larviciding of rivers. More recently it uses mass distribution of ivermectin to complement vector control.

The Onchocerciasis Elimination Programme in the Americas (OEPA) 1991-2007

This regional programme utilises six-monthly mass ivermectin therapy and aims to eliminate clinical manifestations of onchocerciasis and interrupt transmission of disease altogether.

Programme for Onchocerciasis Control (APOC) 1995-2009

This is the largest control programme and comprises large-scale annual distribution of ivermectin in 19 non-OCP countries in Africa. Mectizan® (ivermectin) has been generously donated by Merck and Co. Inc. Caution is needed in areas endemic for both onchocerciasis and loiasis because ivermectin can cause serious adverse effects in patients with high *L. loa* microfilarial loads.

Integrated Control Programmes

Onchocerciasis and lymphatic filariasis commonly co-exist and integrated control programmes employ annual mass treatment of endemic areas with ivermectin and albendazole. GlaxoSmithKline (GSK), formerly SmithKline Beecham, has donated albendazole and Merck and Co Inc expanded their ivermectin donation for lymphatic filariasis control in Yemen and African countries where onchocerciasis and lymphatic filariasis are co-endemic because of the contraindications of DEC in individuals with onchocerciasis.

16.3 LYMPHATIC FILARIASIS

16.3.1 Introduction

Of the 120 million people infected worldwide, 40 million are seriously incapacitated and disfigured. The prevalence of the disease is increasing as unplanned growth of cities creates numerous breeding sites of the mosquito vector.

16.3.2 Clinical picture

Short-term travellers are at low risk for this infection. Travellers to endemic areas for extended periods of time and extensively exposed to mosquitoes may become infected. Most cases seen in developed countries are in immigrants from endemic countries.

Expatriates who are exposed to infection for the first time (e.g. military personnel who are sent to endemic areas) develop acute lymphangitis around developing larval and early adult stages, associated with an eosinophilic inflammatory infiltrate. Newcomers to endemic areas develop acute and chronic manifestations of the disease much more rapidly than residents who have been exposed since birth and lymphedema may develop within six months and elephantiasis within one year of arrival.

Residents of communities endemic for lymphatic filariasis may have 'asymptomatic' infections or develop acute or chronic presentations.

Approximately half of all individuals in endemic areas appear clinically normal but have microfliariae circulating in their blood and have covert lymphatic and renal damage (microscopic haematuria and proteinuria). This state of asymptomatic microfilaria is associated with down-regulation of the immune system.

Acute manifestations

The most common acute problem is 'filarial fevers' affecting the limbs or scrotum which is caused by bacterial or fungal superinfection of tissues with already-compromised lymphatic function. More recently it has been suggested that a better term would be DLA (dermatolymphangioadenitis) to reflect the fact that these inflammatory episodes start peripherally with features resembling cellulitis.

Less frequently, 'filarial fevers' are triggered by an inflammatory response which starts in the lymph node with 'retrograde' extension down the lymphatic tract and an accompanying 'cold' edema.

Tropical pulmonary eosinophilia is a rare syndrome characterized by asthma-type symptoms and often obstructive lung disease. Patients have an immunologic hyper-responsiveness to filarial antigen with high levels of peripheral eosinophilia, total serum IgE and specific IgG and IgE antifilarial antibodies.

Chronic changes

The most common chronic manifestation is hydrocele which increases in prevalence with age. Other chronic manifestations include lymphedema and elephantiasis of the limbs or genitalia and breasts. Such patients are rarely microfilaraemic. The folds, crevices and warty protuberances of an elephantine limb harbour bacteria and fungi which intermittently breach the epidermis and cause local and systemic infection. Chyluria is another chronic presentation.

16.3.3 Diagnostic procedures

Antigen detection

Circulating filarial antigen (CFA) detection should now be regarded as the gold standard for diagnosing *W. bancrofti* infections. It has excellent specificity and greater sensitivity than previous parasite-detection methods and can be used on finger-prick blood samples collected at any time of the day. All individuals with microfilaraemia plus some amicrofilaraemic patients with lymphedema or elephantiasis will have detectable CFA. In addition, some individuals who appear normal also have detectable CFA which disappears after treatment with DEC. Two commercial versions of this assay are available, one based on ELISA technology which yields a semi-quantitative result and the other based on a simple card (immunochromatographic) test which provides a positive/negative result.

Detection of microfilariae by microscopic examination of blood sample

Microfilariae only circulate in the blood at or near the peak biting time of the vector. As the vectors in Africa are all night-biting, blood has to be taken within a few hours either side of midnight, which causes obvious practical problems. Yields may be increased by passing heparinized blood through a Millipore filter, which retains the microfilariae which can then be easily visualised using a microscope. Yields may also be increased by giving 6 mg/kg DEC and repeating the blood film 15 minutes later as DEC releases more microfilariae into the circulation.

PCR diagnosis

Molecular diagnosis using PCR is available for *W. bancrofti* and *B. malayi*.

In the expatriate syndrome, pre-exposure levels of IgG and especially IgG4 antibodies to filarial antigens will be very low, so elevated levels, together with the clinical picture will be helpful diagnostically.

16.3.4 Treatment

DEC

DEC is microfilaricidal and is also effective in killing some, but not all adult worms. For bancroftian filariasis the recommended regime for individual patients is DEC 6 mg/kg daily in divided doses for 12 days. Treatment is best initiated with smaller doses for 2-3 days and antihistamines or corticosteroids may be required to reduce allergic reactions due to disintegration of microfilariae. Combination of treatment with ivermectin (400 µg/kg) is synergistic.

Albendazole can be macrofilaricidal for *W. bancrofti* if given daily for 2-3 weeks. More recently single-dose treatment regimes have been found to be very effective. A single dose combination of albendazole 400 mg with either ivermectin 200 µg/kg or DEC 6 mg/kg can effectively suppress *W. bancrofti* microfilaraemia for a year.

Doxycycline
Doxycycline 200 mg/day for 6 six weeks plus a single dose of ivermectin has been shown to render infected Ghanian residents of an endemic area completely amicro-filaraemic after 12 months (13).

Surgical treatment, including nodo-venous shunts and excision of redundant tissue can improve elephantiasis.

One of the most significant advances in treatment has been the recognition that much of the progressive pathology is due to bacterial and fungal super-infection of tissues with impaired lymphatic function. Rigorous attention to hygiene of affected limbs and measures to improve lymphatic drainage reduce the frequency of 'filarial fevers' and even slowly improve lymphedema and elephantiasis.

16.3.5 Prevention
Protection from mosquito bites through use of personal repellents, bednets or insec-ticide-impregnated materials is prudent. A prophylactic regime of DEC 6 mg/kg per day x 2 days each month may be effective in preventing infection.

The Global Programme for Elimination of Lymphatic Filariasis (GPELF) 1999-2020
This programme aims to eliminate lymphatic filariasis as a public health problem. Covering more than 80 endemic countries, this is the largest mass drug administra-tion programme ever conceived. DEC is used in combination with albendazole out-side Africa and ivermectin plus albendazole is used in Africa, because co-endemicity with onchocerciasis or loiasis prevents use of DEC because of side-effects. Single doses of the two drugs are given together at annual intervals and this needs to be repeated for 4-6 years.

16.4 LOIASIS

16.4.1 Clinical picture
Non-specific symptoms of pruritus, pain or swelling of a limb and urticaria can occur over several months as the fourth-stage larvae develop into adult worms. About a year after infection the characteristic manifestation of loiasis, Calabar swellings, develop.

These are more common in expatriate Europeans and are thought to represent local hypersensitivity reactions to the subcutaneous passage of an adult worm. The swellings, which develop suddenly, are itchy, erythematous, edematous lesions 2-10 cm in diameter and sometimes painful. They can occur anywhere on the skin but are more common on the hand and arm. The swellings slowly resolve over several hours to a few days but can recur. Angioedema may occur and is often more severe in expatriates. The adult worm can sometimes be seen temporarily as it passes across the eye underneath the conjunctiva causing irritation and unilateral palpebral edema, but 'eye-worm' is more common in residents of endemic areas. Other clinical signs include a localised lymphadenopathy, fever, irritability, confusion, epilepsy, orchitis and hydrocele. Nephropathy, cardiomyopathy and pulmonary damage are rare.

16.4.2 Diagnostic procedures

Detection of microfilariae by microscopic examination of day-time blood sample
Microfilariae may be demonstrated in a sample of daytime blood as for *Bancroftian filariasis,* though microfilariae are not found in the blood before about 5 months after the onset of Calabar swellings. *L. loa* microfilariae are sheathed and have nuclei reaching the very end of the tail. Expatriates may have negative peripheral blood examination.

Immunological markers
Infected travellers may have pronounced eosinophilia, high antifilarilal antibodies and positive complement fixation tests using Dirofilarial antigen but these are not specific tests.

Histology
A skin biopsy may sometimes reveal microfilariae in dermal blood vessels.

Molecular diagnosis
Molecular diagnosis is not available yet but a *L.loa*-specific repetitive DNA sequence is known.

16.4.3 Treatment
One course of DEC is usually curative. DEC 1 mg/kg is given as a single dose initially, doubled on 2 successive days and then adjusted to 2-3 mg/kg three times a day for a further 18 days. Rapid killing of microfilariae in heavy infections can provoke an encephalopathy. Prednisolone 20 mg od for 4 days starting one day before DEC may

be given if the patient is microfilaraemic. Albendazole can be used to slowly reduce microfilariae but repeated courses may be necessary.

Ivermectin (200 µg/kg) is also effective but it is not macrofilaricidal. Its use in immigrants from endemic areas, however, may cause an ill-defined encephalopathy in patients with very high *L. loa* microfilarial loads. This poses a problem for mass distribution of ivermectin for onchocerciasis within APOC. Areas which are co-endemic for onchocerciasis and loiasis therefore require careful prior mapping for co-distribution of *Loa loa* so that staff can be appropriately trained in the management of serious reactions and medical supplies obtained.

Wolbachia endosymbionts are absent in *L. loa*.

16.4.4 Prevention
DEC 300 mg weekly may be taken by travellers for as long as exposure continues.

16.5 MANSONELLIASIS

16.5.1 Clinical picture
M. streptocerca can cause pruritus and papular eruptions similar to that seen in onchocerciasis. More widespread lichenification and hypopigmented macules also occur. Infections caused by the two other *Mansonella* species are usually symptomless. *M. perstans* infection can also cause angioedema, pruritus, fever, headaches, arthralgias and neurological problems and *M. ozzardi* can cause a variety of symptoms including pruritus, arthralgias, headaches, fever and lymphadenopathy.

16.5.2 Diagnostic procedures
Microfilariae of all species of *Mansonella* are unsheathed. The features that distinguish microfilariae of *M. streptocerca* from *O. volvulus* are the smaller size of their nuclei and the appearance of their anterior and posterior ends. The cephalic space of *M. streptocerca* microfilariae is longer than it is wide and is followed by a line of 4 staggered but not overlapping elongated nuclei. The tail curves into a characteristic 'shepherd's crook' appearance.

16.5.3 Treatment
DEC, which has activity against both adult worms and microfilariae, may be given at 6 mg/kg per day for 14 days. A single dose of ivermectin 150 µg/kg is microfilaricidal.

REFERENCES
1   Wolfe MS, Petersen JL, Neafie RC, Connor DH, Purtilo DT. Onchocerciasis presenting with swelling of limb. *Am J Trop Med Hyg* 1974;23(3):361-8.

2   Glover M, Murdoch M, Leigh I. Subtle early features of onchocerciasis in a European. *J R Soc Med* 1991;84(7):435.

3   Harvey RJ. The early diagnosis and treatment of onchocerciasis. *Cent Afr J Med* 1967;13(10):242-5.

4   Jopling WH. Onchocerciasis presenting without dermatitis. *Br Med J* 1960;5176:861.

5   Murdoch ME, Hay RJ, Mackenzie CD, Williams JF, Ghalib HW, Cousens S, et al. A clinical classification and grading system of the cutaneous changes in onchocerciasis. *Br J Dermatol* 1993;129(3):260-9.

6   Murdoch ME, Asuzu MC, Hagan M, Makunde WH, Ngoumou P, Ogbuagu KF, et al. Onchocerciasis: the clinical and epidemiological burden of skin disease in Africa. *Ann Trop Med Parasitol* 2002;96(3):283-96.

7   Enk CD, Anteby I, Abramson N, Amer R, Amit Y, Bergshtein-Kronhaus T, et al. Onchocerciasis among Ethiopian immigrants in Israel. *Isr Med Assoc J* 2003;5(7):485-8.

8   Remme JHF. Onchocerciasis. Murray CJL, Lopez AD (eds.). The Global Epidemiology of Infectious Diseases. Cambridge MA, Harvard University Press. Ref Type: Generic.

9   Vlassoff C, Weiss M, Ovuga EB, Eneanya C, Nwel PT, Babalola SS, et al. Gender and the stigma of onchocercal skin disease in Africa. *Soc Sci Med* 2000;50(10):1353-68.

10 Churchill DR, Godfrey-Faussett P, Birley HD, Malin A, Davidson RN, Bryceson AD. A trial of a three-dose regimen of ivermectin for the treatment of patients with onchocerciasis in the UK. *Trans R Soc Trop Med Hyg* 1994;88(2):242.

11 Brieger WR, Awedoba AK, Eneanya CI, Hagan M, Ogbuagu KF, Okello DO, et al. The effects of ivermectin on onchocercal skin disease and severe itching: results of a multicentre trial. *Trop Med Int Health* 1998;3(12):951-61.

12 Hoerauf A, Mand S, Adjei O, Fleischer B, Buttner DW. Depletion of *Wolbachia* endobacteria in *Onchocerca volvulus* by doxycycline and microfilaridermia after ivermectin treatment. *Lancet* 2001;357(9266):1415-6.

13 Hoerauf A, Mand S, Fischer K, Kruppa T, Marfo-Debrekyei Y, Debrah AY, et al. Doxycycline as a novel strategy against bancroftian filariasis-depletion of *Wolbachia* endosymbionts from *Wuchereria bancrofti* and stop of microfilaria production. *Med Microbiol Immunol* (Berl) 2003;192(4):211-6.

17 *Schistosomiasis*

A.M. Polderman

17.1 INTRODUCTION

Schistosomiasis is caused by a number of flukes of the genus *Schistosoma*. The major species involved are *S. mansoni* and *S. japonicum*, which inhabit the venules of the portal and mesenteric system and *S. haematobium* that is found in the venous plexus of the urinogenital system. The characteristic feature of these helminthes is that the adult worms are truly blood parasites but their offspring is excreted with stools or urine of the infected host. Only a part of the eggs produced manages to reach the intestinal lumen or the bladder cavity; many others do not successfully accomplish the migration from veins to intestines and bladder. They die *en route* and are the cause of subsequent pathology, at the predilection sites or elsewhere. The adult worms are of a benign nature and do not normally cause any pathology (1).

17.2 LIFE CYCLE AND EPIDEMIOLOGY

The life cycle of the parasite is complex. It involves a definitive and an intermediate host, two free-living stages, responsible for the infection of humans (cercariae) and snails (miracidia), and both a sexual and an asexual multiplication. The population biology is characterized by the facts that the free-living stages are extremely short-lived (less than 48 hours), the egg-production is low (no more than approximately 300 eggs per gram faeces per day in *S. haematobium* and *S. mansoni*), and the life span is very long. On the average worms are believed to live for 3-5 years but some survive for 30 years or even longer. The essentials of the life cycle of *S. mansoni* are summarized in figure 17.1.

Four different phases of the life cycle each cause a characteristic type of pathology and disease.

1   The penetration of cercariae through the intact human skin may result in so-called cercarial dermatitis or swimmer's itch. This phase is of short duration.
2   The phase of acute schistosomiasis or Katayama syndrome is characterized by a hypersensitivity-type reaction to the excretion of schistosome metabolites into the host's circulation. The onset of this phase may be as early as two weeks post-

exposure; it normally subsides by the time egg excretion starts, 7-10 weeks after the infection.

3 The phase of established infection starts with egg production and may last many years. The symptoms and signs of infection during that stage are caused by the immunopathological host reaction to schistosome eggs that get stuck in the tissues. Sometimes eggs get astray and get stuck in unusual sites: ectopic schistosomiasis may be the result.

4 The final stage can be characterized as the phase of complications due to more or less irreversible fibrotic changes in the periportal and urogenital regions.

Diagnosis varies with the stage of infection and is based on a combination of exposure to surface water in an endemic area, clinical data, stool examination for eggs and serology to determine the presence of specific antibodies. Laboratory diagnosis is complicated by the fact that eggs are not excreted yet in the first two phases of infection. During the phases of established and late chronic infection egg excretion may be very low and eggs are easily missed. Serology is useful in travelers normally living in non-endemic areas, but of little help in endemic regions due to the long persistence of antibodies after clinically successful treatment.

Figure 17.1 Life cycle of S. mansoni (2)

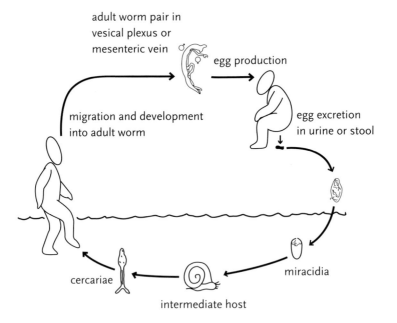

adult worm pair in
vesical plexus or
mesenteric vein

egg production

migration and development
into adult worm

egg excretion
in urine or stool

cercariae

intermediate host

miracidia

Transmission of schistosomiasis is restricted to the tropics and even there the distribution is highly clustered. It is dependent on ecological conditions favourable or unfavourable for the survival and multiplication of the intermediate host snails. The prevalence of infection is often high, particularly in school age children, and is associated with the intensity of exposure to infested water bodies, i.e. with the absence of safe water.

17.3 CLINICAL FEATURES

The most prominent clinical features and the cause of significant morbidity of schistosomiasis in endemic areas are the presence of – sometimes bloody – diarrhea, hepatomegaly and splenomegaly in *S. mansoni* and *S. japonicum* infections and of haematuria in *S. haematobium*. Portal hypertension that is caused by intense granulomatous and fibrotic reactions around eggs that were captured in the liver, hepatomegaly, splenomegaly, and oesophageal and rectal bleeding, mark the late stage of intestinal and hepatosplenic schistosomiasis. The late consequences of *S. haematobium* are related to bladder calcifications and hydronephrosis. All these manifestations are associated with the intensity of infection, i.e. the worm load.

Skin manifestations are not part of these normal clinical features. Yet, they are occasionally seen in infections with all three species of human schistosomes. They are due to cercarial penetration of the human skin, due to the allergic reaction as a component of the Katayama syndrome, and later due to eggs that get astray in situations referred to as cases of ectopic schistosomiasis.

17.3.1 Cercarial dermatitis

The duration of passage through the dermis is normally short. The cercariae loose their tail and the so-called schistosomulae rapidly pass the dermis to be transported to deeper layers. The clinical picture of cercarial dermatitis develops in a matter of minutes, and mostly within one hour after penetration (figure 17.2). In less than a day

Figure 17.2   Swimmer's itch

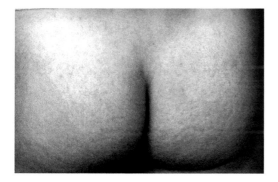

the schistosomulae have passed the skin and reach the lungs; the dermatitis vanishes as well. Mostly this phase of infection is insignificant or absent. In a highly endemic area in Congo I used to be told by the local people that in particular sites exposure to the surface water was unhealthy because it caused itching. In those sites snail and cercarial concentrations were shown to be very high (personal observations). Mostly, however, this phase of infection with the human parasite remains unnoticed by the local population. The situation is different, however, when previously uninfected adults get exposed to (high densities of) cercariae. Intense itching shortly after swimming is commonly described by European or American visitors to endemic countries who are later shown to be infected.

Cercarial dermatitis is much more intense when the cercariae belong to schistosome species unable to successfully infect humans, such as *Ornithobilharzia ocellata* of birds. The schistosomulae of this and related species penetrate the human skin, they migrate through the skin but fail to continue further development to adult worms. After some days they die but meanwhile a much more intense picture of cercarial dermatitis may have developed .

There is no specific means of diagnosis as antibodies haven't been formed yet and eggs can of course not be found either. The roaming schistosomulae cannot normally been recognized. The diagnosis is clinical only and specific therapy is neither indicated nor available (1,3,4).

17.3.2 Urticarial reactions during the Katayama syndrome (Katayama fever)

Urticarial reactivity is generally recognized as a component of the toxaemic phase of infection referred to as the Katayama syndrome. Urticaria, however, are seen in no more than a minority of the Katayama patients. Prostration, fever, profuse sweating and eosinophilia are the accompanying signs of acute schistosome infection. Although originally described for patients with heavy *S. japonicum* infection the Katayama syndrome can be seen in *S. mansoni* and *S. haematobium* patients as well.

Laboratory diagnosis depends on serology but may fail because the antibody responses cannot be measured before day 35 post-infection (5).

17.3.3 Ectopic schistosomiasis

The great majority of migrating schistosomulae efficiently reach their predilection sites in the urogenital system for *S. haematobium*, and in the mesenteric and portal system for *S. mansoni* and *S. japonicum*. It is not amazing that occasionally worms get astray and both adult worms and their eggs get stuck in aberrant sites. Neuroschistosomiasis may result when granulomas develop around eggs in the central nervous system; skin manifestations arise from eggs deposited in the skin.

Ectopic cutaneous schistosomiasis, sometimes referred to as 'bilharziasis cutanea tarda', presents as a papular eruption, sometimes as groups of papules or plaques.

Sometimes they are observed to grow slowly and to form warty or even 'cauliflower projections'. Often but not always the papules are hyperpigmented.

The skin lesions are most frequently found in the perigenital area of female patients. Extragenital skin lesions are seen less frequently. In the cases that have been reported clusters of granulomatous papules have been found on the skin of the trunk, the back, peri-umbilical, and the neck and clavicular regions. Rarely other sites are involved like breasts or limbs.

Anastomoses between the pelvic venous plexus and the subcutaneous plexus of the genitorectal area explain the relative frequency of skin lesions in that area. Those lesions are mostly seen in severe chronic *S. haematobium* infections.

The occurrence of extra-genital lesions cannot be explained in a single straight-forward way. The generally clustered nature of the papules suggests that adult egg-laying worms have been swept into abnormal foci. It has been stated that ectopic localizations of the lesions are a sign of a 'less stable host-parasite relationship'. In this context it is interesting to note that already in 1905, adult egg-laying worms had been found in the lungs of schistosomiasis patients (6). Further evidence for such an unstable host-parasite relationship comes from the observation that many of the extragenital skin lesions are seen shortly after exposure (< 6 months), when the adult worms have hardly settled and started egg production. Young schistosomes require some time to firmly establish in their site of predilection: *S. haematobium* eggs, for instance, are found much more frequently in stool specimens in the early weeks of egg excretion than some months later. In a well-studied case presenting hyper-pigmented lichenoid schistosome papules in the neck of a 12-year-old Nigerian boy, haematuria developed three weeks after presentation of the skin lesions (7). By that time many *S. haematobium* eggs were found in the urine sediment.

The notion of an unbalanced host-parasite relationship to explain the finding of at least some of the ectopic lesions is supported by a number of observations:

1   The papules are consistently found in clusters, indicating that many eggs – and likely egg-laying worms – got astray in the same site.
2   This rare condition is most often found in visitors from non-endemic countries and in children, i.e. in first infections.
3   The time interval between exposure and clinical manifestation is usually (but not always!) short, i.e. less than 6 months.
4   Among the comparatively few cases of extra-genital skin lesions some cases have been seen following treatment failure of a well-established schistosome infection or in association with a presumably schistosome-based transverse myelitis.

Diagnosis of skin lesions is entirely based on the demonstration of schistosome eggs in biopsy specimens. Often eggs are not, or not yet, found in urine or stool specimens. Serological findings support the working hypothesis of a schistosome etiology of the lesion are not a proof (8,9).

17.4 TREATMENT

Praziquantel is the drug of choice for all forms of schistosomiasis. The cure rate of a standard dose of praziquantel (once 40 mg/kg) depends on the worm load but is definitely less than 100%. A somewhat higher dosage or a second treatment might be indicated. Apart from praziquantel to kill the egg producing adult worms additional treatment to cope with abscesses may be needed. In patients with Katayama syndrome, treatment is generally postponed until egg production starts since the drug's efficacy is less targeted at immature stages.

REFERENCES

1   Jordan P, Webbe G, Sturrock RF. Human Schistosomiasis. Wallingford UK: CAB International, 1993:1-465.
2   Polderman AM. Medische Parasitologie. The Netherlands, Oosterbeek: Syntax Media 2005:1-294.
3   Bryceson ADM, Hay RJ. Schistosomiasis, cercarial dermatitis. In: Champion RH, Burton JL, Ebling FGJ (eds.). Textbook of Dermatology, 5th Edition. Oxford/London/Edinburgh/Boston/Melbourne/Paris/Berlin/Vienna: Blackwell Scientific Publications 1992;1237-40.
4   Gentile L de, Picot H, Bourdeau P, Bardet P, Kerjan A, Piriou M, et al. La dermatite cercarienne en Europe: un problème de Santé Publique nouveau? *Bull WHO* 1996;74:159-63.
5   Stuiver PC. Acute Schistosomiasis (Katayama Fever). *Br Med J* 1984;288:221-2.
6   Symmers WSC. A note on a case of bilharzial worms in the pulmonary blood in a case of bilharzial colitis. *Lancet* 1905;I:22.
7   Obasi OE. Cutaneous schistosomiasis in Nigeria. *Br J Dermatol* 1986;114:597-602.
8   Eulderink F, Gryseels B, Kampen WJ van, Regt J de. Haematobium schistosomiasis presenting in the Netherlands as a skin disease. *Am J Dermatopathol* 1994;16(4):434-8.
9   Andrade Filho J de S, Lopes MSSN, Corgozinho Filho AA, Pena GPM. Ectopic cutaneous schistosomiasis: Report of two cases and a review of the literature. *Rev Instit Med Trop Sao Paulo* 1998;40:253-7.

18 Tungiasis

H. Feldmeier and J. Heukelbach

18.1 INTRODUCTION

Tungiasis is a parasitic skin disease due to the permanent penetration of the female sand flea *Tunga penetrans* into the epidermis of its host. Once embedded in the stratum corneum, the flea undergoes a peculiar hypertrophy, during which the abdominal segments enlarge to the size of a pea (called the neosome). Through a tiny opening in the skin hundreds of eggs are expelled for a period of about three weeks (1). After all eggs have been released, the involution of the neosome begins. Three to four weeks after penetration, the parasite dies *in situ* and eventually is sloughed from the epidermis by tissue repair mechanisms.

Tungiasis is known since the 16th century. The first description of the disease was provided by Hans Staden von Homberg zu Hessen, a German adventurer who lived several years with the Tupinambá Indians in an area that nowadays is the State of Rio de Janeiro in Brazil (2).

Being rather rare in travellers, the ectoparasitosis is frequently misdiagnosed and patients are subjected to inappropriate diagnostic and therapeutic procedures.

18.2 EPIDEMIOLOGY: GEOGRAPHIC DISTRIBUTION, MODE OF INFECTION

The sand flea *Tunga penetrans* is one of the few parasites that have spread from the western to the eastern hemisphere. Originally, the ectoparasite occurred only on the American continent. There is anecdotal evidence that the flea came to Angola with ballast sand carried by the ship *Thomas Mitchell* that left from Brazil in 1872. Within a few decades, *T. penetrans* spread from the coast of Angola along trading routes and with advancing troops to vast areas of sub-Saharan Africa. At the end of the 19th century the sand flea had reached East Africa and Madagascar.

Today, tungiasis is found on the American continent from Mexico to northern Argentina, on several Caribbean islands, as well as in almost every country of sub-Saharan Africa (3). A single case report indicates sporadic occurrence in India.

In endemic countries the distribution of tungiasis is uneven and most cases occur in circumscribed foci (3). Typically, these are urban squatter settlements, traditional villages along the coast or underdeveloped communities in the rural hinterland, i.e. places rarely visited by the mainstream tourist.

In economically depressed populations infestation rates are high and prevalences may reach 50% or more (4). Prevalence and parasite burden are related, and in typical foci individuals may harbour between a few and more than 100 fleas. There is a clear seasonality of infestation rates with only few cases occurring during the rainy season and a high incidence during the dry season (5).

Tungiasis is a zoonosis affecting a broad range of domestic and sylvatic animals. For humans dogs, cats, pigs and rats are the most important reservoirs (6).

As the designation 'sand flea' suggests the ectoparasitosis is thought to be associated with sandy soil. However, sand fleas propagate on different types of soil, in the rainforest, in banana plantation and in backyards, provided the ground is covered with some organic material and soil temperature is sufficiently high to allow development from the egg of the adult flea. Infestation may also occur inside a dwelling when the house has no solid floor. Supposedly, infestation may occur at any time of the day. Fleas actively explore the skin in order to probe for a suitable place for penetration. Why in most cases penetration takes places at the feet is not known.

Figure 18.1   Recently penetrated sand flea at the base of a toe. The black dot surrounded by the erythema indicates the abdominal segments of the parasite.

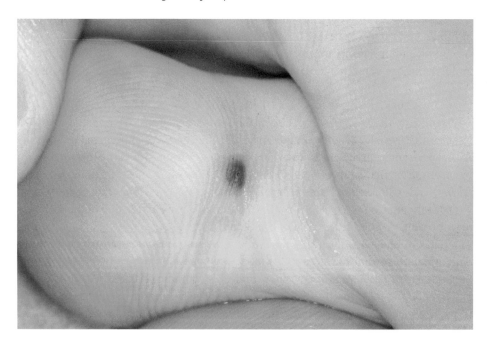

Fleas penetrate the stratum corneum rapidly and are completely burrowed in the epidermis within 30 minutes to several hours (1). The penetration is usually not perceived by the host.

18.3 CLINICAL PICTURE

It is important to understand that tungiasis is a dynamic process with lesions altering their morphological aspect continuously. Hence, the macroscopic appearance of tungiasis in a returned traveller essentially depends on the stage of development of the embedded flea.

Based on clinical and morphological criteria the natural history of tungiasis can be divided into five stages (1). In stage I (flea in *statu penetrandi*, 30 min to several hours) a tiny reddish spot of about 1mm appears with or without an erythematous halo (figure 18.1).

In stage II (beginning hypertrophy with formation of the neosome, one to two days after penetration) the lesion becomes more evident as a growing whitish or mother-of-pearl papule develops. In the protruding rear cone of the flea, the anal-genital opening appears as a central black dot surrounded by erythema (figure 18.2).

Figure 18.2   Lesion in late stage II at the rim of the nail. The circular yellow-whitish area is the neosome which glimmers through the stratum corneum.

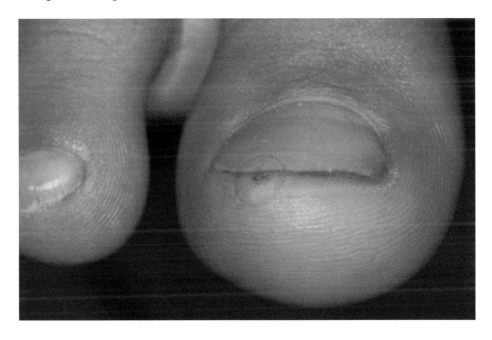

In stage III (maximal hypertrophy, two days to three weeks after penetration) the hypertrophy becomes macroscopically visible. A round, watch glass-like elevation with well-defined borders and tight consistency appears frequently surrounded by local desquamation (figure 18.3).

Emission of eggs and faeces is typical in this stage (figure 18.3 en 18.7). In stage III the lesion is painful and the patient has the sensation of foreign bodies expanding under the skin. In stage IV (three to five weeks after penetration), a black crust covers an involuted lesion with a dead, decaying parasite (figure 18.4).

At the end of stage IV the carcass of the ectoparasite is sloughed from the epidermis leaving a circular depression in the skin. A residual 'scar' in the stratum corneum is characteristic for stage V (six weeks to several months after penetration). Such 'scars' are best seen on the sole (figure 18.5).

Typically, *T. penetrans* affects the periungual area of the toes and the heels. The reason for this is unknown. However, sand fleas can be found on almost every part of the body, e.g. hands, elbows, neck, buttocks and the genital region (7). If several lesions occur simultaneously they are usually located in clusters (figure 18.4 and 18.7). Predilection sites for clusters are the toes, the sole and the heel. In single cases

Figure 18.3   Two lesions at the base of a toe in late stage III and one in late stage II. The distal lesion shows a wrinkled appearance, an indication that regression of the lesion has already begun. Next to the stage II lesion an egg is visible. A fissure has formed below the distal metatarsal joint.

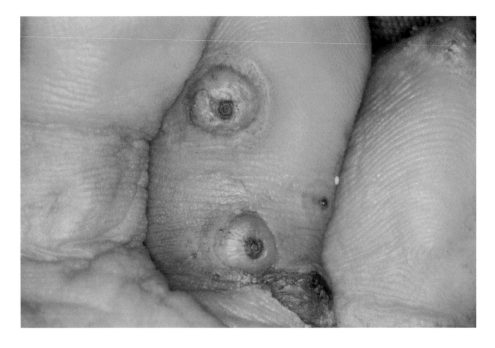

lesions may take the aspect of a tumourous growth and in histological sections appear as a pseudoepitheliomatous hyperplasia (figure 18.6).

The usual sequence, i.e. the development of the neosome, involution of the lesion and 'scar' formation may be changed by two events: superinfection and manipulation of the lesion by the patient or his carer.

In the endemic area superinfection is present in virtually all cases as the development of the lesion progresses (8). In tourists superinfection is less common. Superinfection first leads to the formation of a micro abscess, then to a pustule and eventually to suppuration (figure 18.7).

Staphylococcus aureus and streptococci are the micro-organisms most frequently responsible, but other aerobic and anaerobic bacteria (including clostridiae) are also found (8). In non-vaccinated individuals tungiasis may lead to tetanus. Pathogenic micro-organisms or their toxins reach deeper layers of the skin (and finally also the circulation), because the outer surface of the skin is linked to the dermis by the body of the ectoparasite of which the proboscis is placed in capillaries of the dermis.

If the flea is completely taken out with a sharp instrument during maximal hypertrophy, a visible ulcer remains which easily becomes superinfected. If the ectoparasite ruptures during manipulation – or the mouth part remains embedded at the epidermal-dermal interface – an intense inflammation ensues.

Figure 18.4   Cluster of lesions at the base of the fifth toe surrounded by pus. Lesions are covered by a black crust and sand fleas presumably already died in situ.

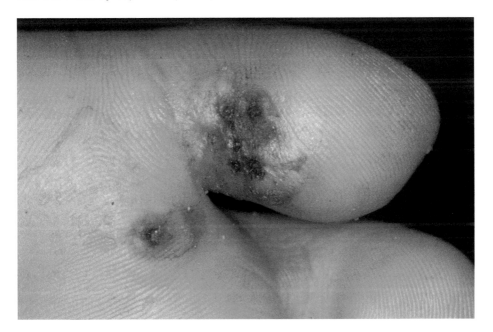

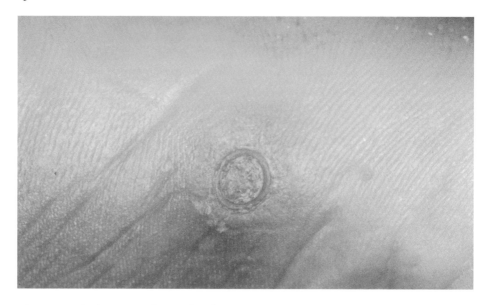

Figure 18.5   Circular 'scar' at the rim of the foot. A sand flea was embedded here several weeks ago. The circular band shows the diameter of skin tissue which had been displaced by the neosome.

Figure 18.6   Unusual aspect of tungiasis at the navel of a child. The tumourous growth is caused by several sand fleas embedded closely to each other.

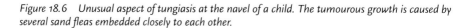

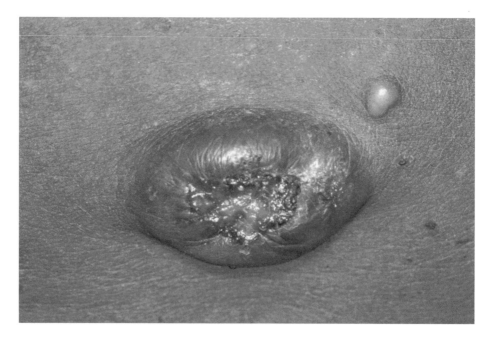

18.4 DIAGNOSIS

The diagnosis is made clinically taking into consideration the dynamic nature of the macroscopic appearance of the lesion together with the geographical history of the patient. The use of a dermatoscope is very helpful. The patient typically complains about local itching, pain and the sensation of a foreign body. The simultaneous presence of two or more identical lesions at the toes, particularly along the nail rim, is diagnostic. The observation of eggs being expelled or attached to the skin around the lesion and the release of brownish threads of faeces are pathognomonic signs (figure 18.3 and 18.7). Faeces threads are of a helical structure and often spread into the dermal papillae. Expulsion of eggs can be provoked by massaging the hypertrophy zone slightly.

The differential diagnosis differs according to the stage. Important differential diagnoses are summarised in table 18.1.

Biopsy of the lesion followed by a histopathological examination is not indicated except in lesions with a pseudoepitheliomatous appearance. Histological sections usually demonstrate the presence of the ectoparasite or of chitinous fragments.

Figure 18.7   A cluster of three lesions at the rim of the nail. Two faecal threads are located left to the cluster. One faecal thread is being ejected. Faecal material is spread in dermal papillae.

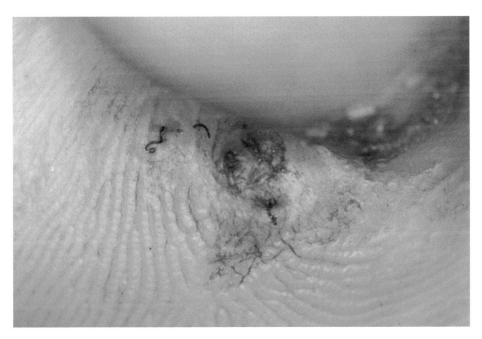

Table 18.1   Differential diagnosis of tungiasis according to stage

Stage	Differential diagnosis	Indicators of tungiasis
I	partially penetrated foreign body (e.g. thorn)	itching, developing erythema, flea disappears completely in the skin with several hours
II	foreign body; insect sting; acute paronychia	itching; circular whitish, mother-of-pearl papule increasing in size with a central black dot; untypical location for insect stings (e.g. nail rim)
III	myiasis; dermoid cyst; wart; pustule/abscess of bacterial origin; dracontiasis	circular watch-glass like elevation with a tight consistency surrounded by desquamation; lesion diameter increases from day to day; expulsion of eggs; expulsion of faecal threads; faecal material dispersed in dermal papillae; sharp localized pain; dracontiasis usually located on the instep or above the ankles
IV	local gangrene, melanoma	development of black crust within a couple of days; rear cone of flea visible in the centre of the black crust; size of lesion gets smaller from day to day

18.5 TREATMENT AND PREVENTION

Surgical extraction of the flea under sterile conditions is the appropriate treatment. The opening in the epidermis must be widened, e.g. with a scalpel, until the neosome is completely liberated from the covering stratum corneum. Then the entire flea has to be carefully taken out with tweezers. After the extraction of the parasite, the wound should be treated with a topical antibiotic. The tetanus immune status has to be checked.

Closed shoes and socks protect to a certain degree against invading fleas. Daily inspection of the feet and immediate extraction of embedded fleas prevents against complications. The twice-daily application of Zanzarin®, a plant-based repellent against culicidae and ticks, reduced the infestation rate in an area with extremely high transmission rates by almost 90 percent (9).

REFERENCES

1   Eisele M, Heukelbach J, Marck E van, Mehlhorn H, Meckes O, Francks S, Feldmeier H. Investigations on the biology, epidemiology, pathology and control of Tunga penetrans in Brazil: I. Natural history of tungiasis in man. *Parasitol Res* 2003;90:87-99.

2   Staden von Homberg zu Hessen H. Wahrhaftige Historia und Beschreibung einer Landschaft der wilden, nacketen, grimmigen Menschenfresser Leuten, in der Neuen Welt America gelegen. Frankfurt am Main: Weigand Hahn, 1556.

3   Heukelbach J, Oliveira FA de, Hesse G, Feldmeier H. Tungiasis: a neglected health problem of poor communities. *Trop Med Int Health* 2001;6:267-72.

4   Muehlen M, Heukelbach J, Wilcke T, Winter B, Mehlhorn H, Feldmeier H. Investigations on the biology, epidemiology, pathology and control of *Tunga penetrans* in Brazil II. Prevalence, parasite load and topographic distribution of lesions in the population of a traditional fishing village. *Parasitol Res* 2003;90,449-55.

5   Heukelbach J, Wilcke T, Harms G, Feldmeier H. Seasonal variation of tungiasis in an endemic community. *Am J Trop Med Hyg* 2005;72:154-9.

6   Heukelbach J, Costa ALM, Wilcke T, Mencke N, Feldmeier H. The animal reservoir of *Tunga penetrans* in poor communities in Northeast Brazil. *Med Vet Entomol* 2004;18:329-35.

7   Heukelbach J, Wilcke T, Eisele M, Feldmeier H. Ectopic localization of tungiasis. *Am J Trop Med Hyg* 2002;67:214-6.

8   Feldmeier H, Heukelbach J, Eisele M, Sousa AO, Barboza LM, Carvalho CB. Bacterial superinfection in human tungiasis. *Trop Med Int Health* 2002;7:559-64.

9   Feldmeier H, Kehr D, Heukelbach H. A plant-based repellent protects against *T. penetrans* and sand flea disease. *Acta Tropica* in press.

19 Creeping eruption (cutaneous larva migrans)

J. Heukelbach and H. Feldmeier

19.1 INTRODUCTION

Creeping eruption (cutaneous larva migrans; plumber's itch; duck hunter's itch) is a parasitic skin disease caused by the penetration of larvae – most commonly of dog and cat hookworms – into the epidermis of humans (1). In the human host, the larvae cannot complete their life cycle and develop into adult worms. They continue migrating in the epidermis for a limited period of time after which they die, disintegrate and are resolved by skin repair mechanisms. The characteristic clinical picture is a pruritic and serpiginous lesion. The larva visibly moves in the skin from day to day.

Cutaneous larva migrans is the most common dermatological problem in travellers returning from tropical and subtropical areas (2). The first description of creeping eruption dates back to 1874 (3). Fifty-five years later, the dermatosis was attributed to animal hookworms (4).

19.2 EPIDEMIOLOGY: GEOGRAPHIC DISTRIBUTION, MODE OF INFECTION

The dog and cat hookworm *Ancylostoma braziliense* is the most common cause, but other species can also cause the infestation, such as the dog hookworm *Ancylostoma caninum*, *Gnathostoma spinigerum* or *Uncinaria stenocephala* (5). Nematodes of other animals such as sheep, goat, cattle and sylvatic animals may also cause creeping eruption. The human nematode *Strongyloides stercoralis*, more commonly associated with a similar syndrome known as larva currens, causes cutaneous larva migrans in single cases.

Creeping eruption is common in tropical and subtropical regions throughout the world. In typical endemic areas in developing countries, a high proportion of dogs and cats are infected with animal hookworms. Animal faeces are spread by heavy rains, and eggs are distributed over a large surface. First stage larvae hatch from eggs within some days after faeces have been deposited. About seven days later, larvae develop in the soil into the infective third stage and are able to penetrate into the epidermis of its host. In a warm and humid environment, where larvae are protected from direct sunlight and desiccation, they can survive for several months. As in resource-poor communities many people walk barefoot and children crawl or sit naked on the ground, prevalence of creeping eruption may be as high as 3% in the general population (6).

Most cases of creeping eruption seen by physicians in industrialized countries are travellers returning from the tropics and subtropics (7,8,9). However, infestation occurs sporadically also in temperate zones, and cases have been described e.g. in the United States, Great Britain, Germany and New Zealand (10).

The infestation of man with animal hookworms occurs accidentally. Individuals become infested when the skin has been in contact with contaminated soil containing larvae of animal hookworms. In contrast to human hookworms these larvae cannot penetrate the basal membrane and therefore remain sequestered in the epidermis. As man is a dead end, the disease is self-limiting. In the epidermis, the larvae migrate aimlessly for a period of weeks and in single cases up to several months causing the pathognomonic clinical picture of creeping eruption.

Travellers typically get infested at the beach of tropical and subtropical countries which are contaminated with dog and cat faeces. The infestation can also be acquired at any place where unprotected skin comes into contact with soil contaminated by animal faeces, such as sand boxes, construction sites and crawl spaces under houses.

Figure 19.1   Creeping eruption: a single serpiginous track

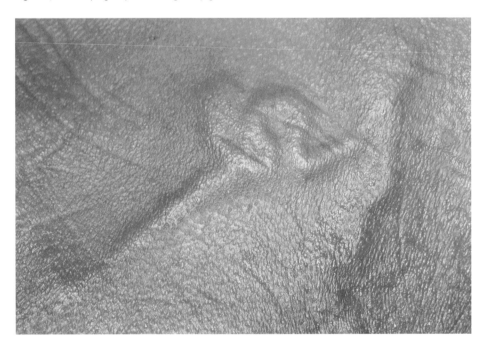

Rarely, infestation occurs via fomites, such as towels or clothes that came into contact with soil while drying.

In tourists, walking barefoot to and on the beach has been the only risk factor identified so far (11).

19.3 CLINICAL PICTURE

Cutaneous larva migrans begins with a reddish papule at the penetration site a few hours after contact with the infective larva. One to several days after penetration, the characteristic erythematous serpiginous, slightly elevated track appears which with time may reach more than 20cm (figure 19.1 and figure 19.2). Depending on the hookworm species, larvae migrate some millimetres up to a few centimetres per day.

Creeping eruption is accompanied by intense itching impeding patients from sleeping normally. The pruritus is generally more intense at night, and patients consider the condition as extremely uncomfortable, particularly when several eruptions are present simultaneously.

Pain may be present. Secondary infection is common and a result of scratching. Sporadically, larvae may invade the viscera and cause eosinophilic pneumonia (Loef-

Figure 19.2   Larval track on the hand of a two-year old girl

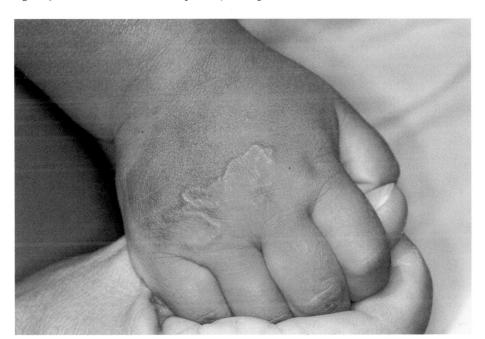

fler's syndrome). Vesiculo-bullous lesions are observed in 9-15% of cases (figure 19.3) (2,8).

Erythema multiforme is rarely seen as a complication in previously sensitized individuals. Folliculitis has been described in single cases.

In travellers, lesions are usually located on the feet, buttocks and thighs, areas which come into contact with contaminated sand while walking or sitting on the beach (7,8,9,12). Rarely, lesions are found also on the arms, elbows, legs, knees and back. In fact, creeping eruption may occur at any topographical site of the body including the face, the oral cavity and the genitals (figures 19.4, 19.5 and 19.6) (6). Patients may have multiple tracks affecting different topographical sites.

19.4 DIAGNOSIS

The diagnosis of creeping eruption is based upon the characteristic clinical picture together with a travel history in which the patient remembers contact with soil. The infestation can be diagnosed by the naked eye. An elevated linear or serpiginous lesion, with or without an erythematous papule (the latter indicating the entry site of the larva) associated with pruritus is pathognomonic. A biopsy is not indicated and – if done – almost never reveals a positive result; the anterior end of the track does

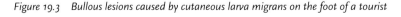

Figure 19.3   Bullous lesions caused by cutaneous larva migrans on the foot of a tourist

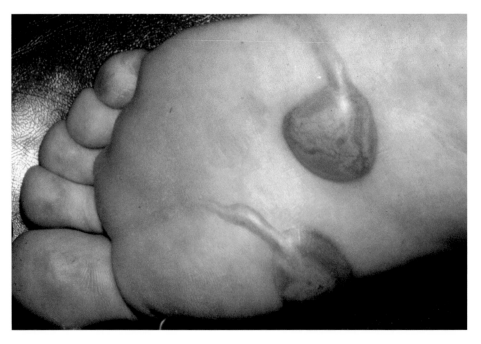

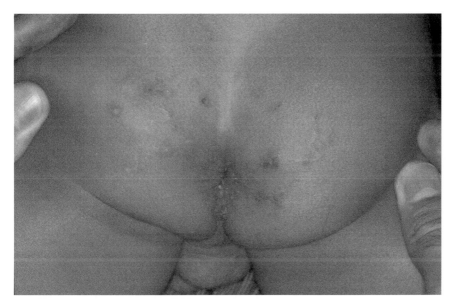

Figure 19.4   Creeping eruption on the buttocks and perianal area of a boy. Several larval tracks can be seen.

Figure 19.5   Multiple creeping eruptions in the genital area of a two-year old girl

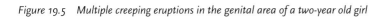
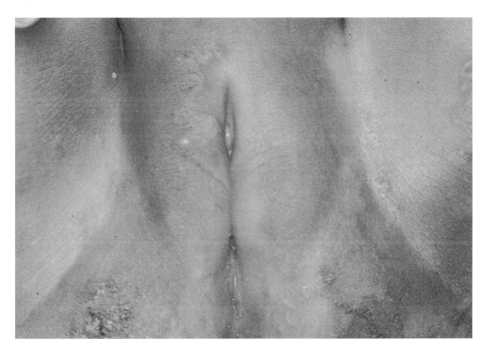

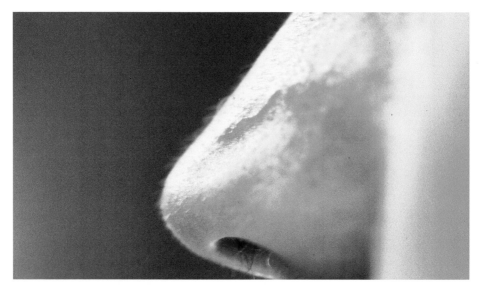

Figure 19.6   Creeping eruption on the nose of a tourist. Infestation occurred by a contaminated towel that had fallen on the ground. Other sites infested were the buttocks, the knee, the scrotum and the arm.

Figure 19.7   Sign prohibiting the presence of dogs on a beach in Brazil as a means of prevention

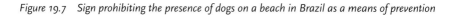

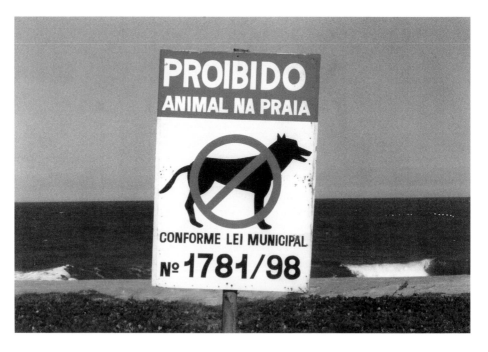

not necessarily indicate the localization of the larva, as the inflammatory response may be delayed.

Laboratory investigations are not helpful. Eosinophilia may or may not be present.

As a differential diagnosis larva currens has to be considered, which is caused by auto-infection with *S. stercoralis*. Larvae of *S. stercoralis* migrate faster than those of animal hookworms (up to several centimetres per hour) and lesions usually start in the perianal area, from where they move towards the abdomen.

Cutaneous gnathostomiasis caused most commonly by the nematode *Gnathostoma spinigerum* is endemic in Southeast Asia, but occurs also in Latin America. It is acquired by eating uncooked fish, frogs or flesh from other animals containing encysted larvae. The third stage larvae migrate in the skin and subcutaneous tissue, but may also enter the central nervous system and other organs. The disease is characterized by itching migratory subcutaneous swellings and creeping eruption-like migration of larvae in the skin. Often, the patients have general symptoms such as headache and fatigue.

Other differential diagnoses include scabies, loiasis, myiasis, cercarial dermatitis (induced by various types of schistosomes), superficial mycosis (tinea), herpes zoster and contact dermatitis.

19.5 TREATMENT AND PREVENTION

The drug of choice is ivermectin. A single dose of oral ivermectin (200 µg/kg) kills the larvae and resolves the symptoms quickly (13). Treatment failure is rare and usually resolves after a second dose. Ivermectin has been used in millions of individuals in the developing world during onchocerciasis and filariasis control operations without any significant adverse events. The drug is contraindicated in children < 15 kg (or < 5 years of age) and pregnant/breastfeeding women. Oral albendazole (400 mg daily for three days) shows also excellent cure rates and is a good alternative for ivermectin. Thiabendazole ointment (10-15%) applied to affected areas three times daily for seven days is as effective as the oral treatment, but requires a substantial compliance from the patient. Oral thiabendazole should be avoided as it is not well tolerated and has considerable side effects such as headache, nausea and dizziness. Freezing the edge of the track with liquid nitrogen or carbon dioxide is obsolete, as it is ineffective, painful and may cause ulcerations.

Secondary infections should be treated with a topical antibiotic.

To prevent infestation of tourists, animals should be banned from beaches (figure 19.7).

The only means of prevention on individual level is avoiding that unprotected skin comes into contact with possibly contaminated ground. This can be achieved by wearing shoes while walking on beaches in endemic areas and not lying directly on the sand at beaches or greens where dogs or cats have been observed. Lying on towels does not protect sufficiently, and a sun chair or mattress should be used. Areas where the sand is humidified by the tide are safe. Towels and clothes should not touch the ground when hung up for drying. In general, places where dogs and cats stroll around should be avoided.

REFERENCES

1   Heukelbach J, Feldmeier H. Ectoparasites – the underestimated realm. *Lancet* 2004;13;363(9412):889-91.

2   Caumes E, Carriere J, Guermonprez G, Bricaire F, Danis M, Gentilini M. Dermatoses associated with travel to tropical countries: a prospective study of the diagnosis and management of 269 patients presenting to a tropical disease unit. *Clin Infect Dis* 1995;20(3):542-8.

3   Lee RJ. Case of creeping eruption. *Trans Clin Soc London* 1874;8:44-5.

4   White GF, Dove WE. A dermatitis caused by larvae of *Ancyolostoma caninum*. *Arch Dermatol* 1929;20:191-200.

5   Beaver PC. Larva migrans. *Exp Parasitol* 1956;5:587-621.

6   Heukelbach J, Wilcke T, Meier A, Saboia Moura RC, Feldmeier H. A longitudinal study on cutaneous larva migrans in an impoverished Brazilian township. *Travel Med Infect Dis* 2003;1(4):213-8.

7   elinek T, Maiwald H, Nothdurft HD, Loscher T. Cutaneous larva migrans in travelers: synopsis of histories, symptoms, and treatment of 98 patients. *Clin Infect Dis* 1994;19(6):1062-6.

8   Davies HD, Sakuls P, Keystone JS. Creeping eruption. A review of clinical presentation and management of 60 cases presenting to a tropical disease unit. *Arch Dermatol* 1993;129(5):588-91.

9   Bouchaud O, Houze S, Schiemann R, Durand R, Ralaimazava P, Ruggeri C et al. Cutaneous larva migrans in travelers: A prospective study, with assessment of therapy with ivermectin. *Clin Infect Dis* 2000;31(2):493-8.

10 Diba VC, Whitty CJ, Green T. Cutaneous larva migrans acquired in Britain. *Clin Exp Dermatol* 2004;29(5):555-6.

11 Tremblay A, MacLean JD, Gyorkos T, Macpherson DW. Outbreak of cutaneous larva migrans in a group of travellers. *Trop Med Int Health* 2000;5(5):330-4.

12 Blackwell V, Vega-Lopez F. Cutaneous larva migrans: clinical features and management of 44 cases presenting in the returning traveller. *Br J Dermatol* 2001;145(3):434-7.

13 Caumes E. Treatment of cutaneous larva migrans and Toxocara infection. *Fundam Clin Pharmacol* 2003;17(2):213-6.

20 Myiasis

D.A. Burns

20.1 **INTRODUCTION**

Myiasis (derived from the Greek *myia* = a fly) is a term used to denote infestation of the body tissues of humans and animals by the larvae (maggots) of flies (Diptera). As an infestation of animals it has enormous economic impact. Human myiasis is often encountered in parts of the tropics, but is uncommon in temperate zones. However, increasing holiday travel and student meanderings during gap years means that practitioners working in non-endemic areas may encounter imported myiasis.

In one study of patients presenting to a tropical disease unit in Paris myiasis was the fourth most common travel-associated disease (1).

There are various forms of myiasis, and several classifications have been proposed in the past (2,3,4,5). Essentially, myiasis may be classified according to parasitological criteria (based on the type of host-parasite relationship) or clinical criteria (the part of the host's body infested) (table 20.1).

Parasitologically, myiasis-producing flies may be subdivided into two principal groups: 'facultative' and 'obligatory'. Larvae of facultative myiasis producers usually develop on decaying flesh or vegetable matter, but may infest wounds. However, it is necessary for obligatory myiasis producers to pass their larval stage parasitically in the body of an animal. Occasionally, larvae are found in the human intestinal or urinary tracts. In such so-called 'accidental' myiasis (also known as pseudomyiasis) the larvae are not living parasitically but have been inadvertently ingested with food, or have wandered into these areas. There is no dipterous obligate intestinal parasite of humans.

Clinically, myiasis can be classified according to the part of the body affected. Cutaneous myiasis includes wound myiasis, in which larvae are present in open wounds and sores, and migratory and furuncular myiasis. Migratory myiasis is similar to cutaneous larva migrans, in that larvae wander in the skin, and in furuncular myiasis the presence of the larvae is associated with boil-like lesions. All species responsible for furuncular myiasis are obligatory parasites. In nasopharyngeal myiasis,

Table 20.1   Principal flies causing cutaneous myiasis in humans

	Parasitic type	Type of myiasis
Calliphoridae		
Chrysoma bezziana	*obligatory*	*wound*
Cochliomyia hominivorax	*obligatory*	*wound*
Cordylobia anthropophaga	*obligatory*	*furuncular*
Cordylobia rodhaini	*obligatory*	*furuncular*
Phormia	*facultative*	*wound*
Lucilia	*facultative*	*wound*
Calliphora	*facultative*	*wound*
Sarcophagidae		
Sarcophaga	*facultative*	*wound*
Wohlfahrtia magnifica	*obligatory*	*wound*
Wohfahrtia vigil	*obligatory*	*furuncular*
Wohlfahrtia opaca	*obligatory*	*furuncular*
Oestridae		
Cuterebra	*obligatory*	*furuncular*
Dermatobia	*obligatory*	*furuncular*
Gasterophilus	*obligatory*	*migratory*
Hypoderma	*obligatory*	*migratory and furuncular*
Muscidae		
Fannia canicularis	*facultative*	*wound*
Musca domestica	*facultative*	*wound*

the nose, sinuses and pharynx are affected, ophthalmomyiasis involves the eye, orbit and periorbital tissues, and in otomyiasis larvae are present in the ear – for example in neglected chronic suppurative otitis media.

20.2 MYIASIS-PRODUCING DIPTERA, GEOGRAPHICAL DISTRIBUTION AND MODE OF INFECTION

The flies responsible for myiasis in humans include the following families.

Calliphoridae (blowflies)

Genus Chrysoma

Chrysoma bezziana, the Old World screwworm, is important medically because the larvae are obligate parasites in wounds. It occurs throughout much of Africa, India, the Arabian peninsula, southeast Asia and the Indonesian and Philippine islands to New Guinea.

Genus Cochliomyia

The New World screwworm *Cochliomyia hominivorax* (previously known as *Cochliomyia americana* and *Callitroga americana*) is an obligate parasite of cattle and other livestock in the Americas. The species name 'human-eater' was coined after larvae from this fly were thought to be associated with the deaths of hundreds of prisoners on Devil's Island (6). It is no longer established in North America, following intensive eradication efforts involving the release of huge numbers of sterile male flies.

Larvae of *C. hominivorax* feed on living tissue, and can penetrate unbroken skin, but they may also infest wounds.

Cochliomyia macellaria can cause myiasis in humans, usually in immobile and debilitated individuals.

Genus Cordylobia

Cordylobia anthropophaga, the tumbu fly, a cause of furuncular myiasis, is widespread in tropical Africa south of the Sahara. Although most reported cases of tumbu fly myiasis are acquired in Africa, there are a few reports of myiasis acquired elsewhere, and it is possible that some of these might be related to contact with eggs on clothing transported from endemic areas.

Cordylobia rodhaini (also known as Lund's fly), the only other species of *Cordylobia* known to infest humans, has a more limited distribution in tropical Africa, principally the rainforest areas. In most cases there is more than one lesion, and very extensive furuncular myiasis due to *C. rodhaini*, acquired in Ethiopia, has been reported in an Italian man.

Eggs are laid on sand or soil, especially if contaminated by urine or faeces, and also on laundry hanging out to dry. In the wild, rats are the usual host, but around human habitation dogs and humans are common hosts. The larva attaches itself to the host by means of its oral hooks, and rapidly penetrates the skin. When development is complete (usually in 14-16 days) it leaves the host and falls to the ground to pupate.

Other genera

Larvae of members of the genera *Phormia* (black blowflies), *Lucilia* (*Phaenicia*) (greenbottle), and *Calliphora* (bluebottle) may also be secondary invaders of wounds in humans. In a recent study of wound myiasis in urban and suburban USA (in which homelessness, alcoholism and peripheral vascular disease were frequent cofactors) the majority of species identified were blowflies, the most common being *Lucilia sericata* (6).

There has been a recent resurgence of interest in the use of maggots for wound debridement, and the larvae of *Lucilia sericata* are used for this purpose (7).

Sarcophagidae (flesh flies)

Genus Sarcophaga
Wound infestation by members of this genus has been reported.

Genus Wohlfahrtia
Similar to *Sarcophaga*, and a cause of wound myiasis. Female flies deposit larvae in wounds or beside body orifices. They are important obligate myiasis-producing flies in camels and sheep. The larvae of *Wohlfahrtia magnifica* may be deposited in the ear, eye and nose, and can cause extensive destruction of healthy tissue. *W. magnifica* occurs throughout the Mediterranean basin, east and central Europe and Asia Minor.

W. vigil and *W. opaca* are North American species whose females deposit larvae on the skin of young animals, resulting in furuncular myiasis. Human furuncular myiasis from these species occurs only in infants, as the larvae are unable to penetrate adult skin.

Oestridae
The Oestridae are all obligate parasites.

Genus Cuterebra (rodent or rabbit botfly)
Rabbits and rodents are the natural hosts for the larvae of these flies, which are sometimes responsible for human furuncular myiasis in North America (8).

Genus Dermatobia (human botfly)
Dermatobia hominis is the only species in the genus. It is a bluebottle-like fly found in the neotropical areas of the New World, extending from southern Mexico to northern Argentina. It occurs where temperature and humidity are relatively high, principally in lowland forests. *D. hominis* causes cutaneous myiasis in a wide range of mammalian hosts, including humans, and is particularly important as a parasite of cattle.

The female fly does not deposit her eggs directly on the host, but uses other insects such as day-flying mosquitoes and blood-sucking flies, as vectors to carry her eggs to the host (a process known as phoresy). She grabs the insect vector in mid-air and deposits a number of eggs on its abdomen. When the vector subsequently feeds on a potential host the eggs hatch and the larvae rapidly burrow into the skin. Larval development lasts approximately 50-60 days, following which the larva emerges, drops to the ground and pupates. Persistent boil-like lesions in anyone who has returned from an endemic area should always raise suspicions of botfly myiasis (9,10).

Genus Gasterophilus (horse botfly)

A form of migratory cutaneous myiasis known as 'creeping eruption' is caused by *Gasterophilus* larvae. These botflies are principally parasites of the alimentary tract of horses, but occasionally larvae of certain species, including G. *haemorrhoidalis* and G. *pecorum*, penetrate human skin.

Genus Oestrus (sheep nostril fly)

Oestrus ovis, which develops in the nasopharyngeal passages of sheep and goats, and *Rhinoestrus purpureus*, which parasitizes horses and donkeys, are occasionally responsible for human myiasis, especially ophthalmomyiasis.

Genus Hypoderma (warble flies)

The larvae of *Hypoderma* species are obligate parasites of cattle. Humans are abnormal hosts, and the larvae do not mature fully. After penetrating the skin the larvae produce migratory subcutaneous swellings. Systemic illness, with myositis, pleurisy and pericarditis, and marked eosinophilia, may accompany infestation.

Muscidae

Fannia canicularis (lesser house fly) and *Musca domestica* (house fly) may deposit their eggs in wounds and ulcers, giving rise to facultative wound myiasis.

20.3 CLINICAL FEATURES

The habits of the flies and their larvae are the principal factors that determine the clinical manifestations for which they are responsible. Facultative wound myiasis is a complication of war wounds in tropical areas, and is an occasional occurrence in most parts of the world, particularly during hot weather when wounds or ulcers are exposed. The larvae (maggots) can be seen, sometimes in large numbers, in the suppurating tissues, and their removal of necrotic tissue and beneficial effect on granulation has led to their use in maggot debridement therapy.

Obligatory cutaneous myiasis occurs in two main clinical forms, and may be accompanied by mild constitutional symptoms and eosinophilia. Both forms occur more commonly on exposed skin, but any site, including the genitalia, may be affected. In the furuncular form, boil-like lesions develop gradually over a few days. Each lesion has a central punctum, which discharges serosanguinous fluid. The posterior end of the larva, equipped with a group of spiracles (figure 20.1 A), is usually visible in the punctum, and its movements are usually noticed by the patient. The lesions are often extremely painful. The inflammatory reaction around the lesions may be accompanied by lymphangitis and regional lymphadenopathy. Once the larva has emerged, or has been removed, the lesions rapidly resolve. The flies causing furuncular myiasis in humans are *Dermatobia hominis*, *Cuterebra* species, *Cordylobia anthropophaga* and *Cordylobia rodhaini*, and *Wohlfahrtia* species.

The second principal clinical form is a creeping eruption, in which there is either a tortuous, thread-like red line with a terminal vesicle (*Gasterophilus*), where the larva lies ahead of the vesicle in apparently normal skin, or a series of inflammatory nodular lesions (*Hypoderma*). *Hypoderma* species also produce furuncular lesions.

20.4 DIAGNOSIS

Diagnosis of furuncular myiasis is usually straightforward – based on a history of a visit to an endemic area and the presence of boil-like lesions in which the patient is aware of movement. However, ultrasonography can facilitate diagnosis and assist in location of the larvae (11).

It is important to precisely identify any larvae recovered in cases of myiasis as this will enable determination of whether they are facultative or obligatory parasites, and thereby their pathogenic potential. The help of an entomologist with special knowledge of Diptera should be sought.

20.5 TREATMENT

The larvae of furuncular myiasis-producers can often be expressed by firm pressure around the edges of the lesions, but the punctum may require enlarging surgically.

However, the larva of *Dermatobia hominis* has a bulbous anterior end equipped with rows of backward-pointing spines (figure 20.1 B and 20.1 C), and cannot easily be expressed because of these. Traditional methods of treatment include occluding the punctum with pork fat, which blocks the spiracles of the larva and stimulates premature extrusion. A similar result may be obtained with mineral oil, petrolatum or butter. Surgical management involves enlargement of the punctum by cruciate incisions that enable removal of an intact larva (figure 20.1 D).

The injection of lidocaine beneath the nodule may be sufficient to push the larva out, and injection of lidocaine into the blind end of the cavity is also said to facilitate its non-surgical removal. In addition, a commercial venom extractor has also proved effective in removing a *D. hominis* larva (figure 20.2).

Wound myiasis requires debridement and irrigation to remove larvae, and treatment of secondary infection.

Topical ivermectin has been used in wound myiasis caused by *C. hominivorax*, and oral ivermectin has been employed in the management of cavitory myiasis, where manual removal of larvae would be painful and unpleasant, and also in infestation with *Hypoderma* (12).

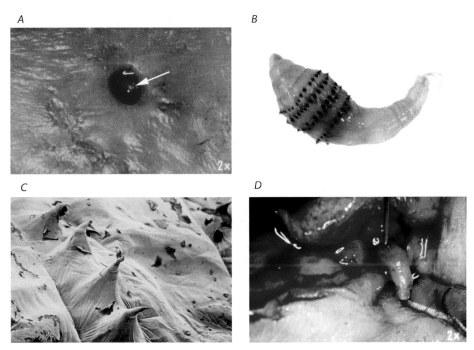

Figure 20.1   (A) Boil-like lesion occupied by Dermatobia hominis larva (arrow), acquired in Belize. The
larva of D. hominis has a bulbous anterior end, equipped with rows of backward-pointing hooks, which
prevent its easy removal from the cavity it occupies (B and C). The punctum has been enlarged by cruciate incisions, and the larva is being removed (D).

Anyone travelling to endemic areas should receive advice appropriate to the area,
including use of insect repellents, the wearing of suitable clothing to cover the limbs,
and ironing of any clothing that has been hung out to dry before it is worn.

Figure 20.2   Lesion on the chin (A) occupied by D. hominis larva (B)

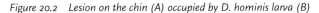

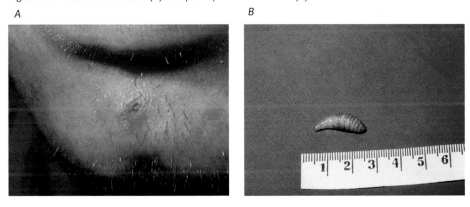

REFERENCES

1   Caumes E, Carrière J, Guermonprez G, Bricaire F, Danis M, Gentilini M. Dermatoses associated with travel to tropical countries: a prospective study of the diagnosis and management of 269 patients presenting to a tropical disease unit. *Clin Infect Dis* 1995;20:542-8.

2   Zumpt F. Myiasis in Man and Animals in the Old World. London: Butterworths, 1965.

3   Alexander JO'D. Arthropods and Human Skin. Berlin: Springer Verlag, 1984:87-113.

4   Hall MJR, Smith KGV. Diptera causing myiasis in man. In: Lane RP, Crosskey RW (eds.). Medical Insects and Arachnids. London: Chapman and Hall, 1993:429-69.

5   Hall M, Wall R. Myiasis of humans and domestic animals. *Adv Parasitol* 1995;35:257-334.

6   Sherman RA. Wound myiasis in urban and suburban United States. *Arch Intern Med* 2000;160:2004-14.

7   Sherman RA, Hall MJR, Thomas S. Medicinal maggots: an ancient remedy for some contemporary afflictions. *Annu Rev Entomol* 2000;45:55-81.

8   Baird JK, Baird CR, Sabrosky CW. North American cuterebrid myiasis. *J Am Acad Dermatol* 1989;21:763-72.

9   Gordon PM, Hepburn NC, Williams AE, Bunney MH. Cutaneous myiasis due to *Dermatobia hominis*: a report of six cases. *Br J Dermatol* 1995;132:811-4.

10 Maier H, Hönigsmann H. Furuncular myiasis caused by *Dermatobia hominis*, the human botfly. *J Am Acad Dermatol* 2004;50:S26-30.

11 Bowry R, Cottingham RL. Use of ultrasound to aid management of late presentation of *Dermatobia hominis* larva infestation. *J Accid Emerg Med* 1997;14:177-86.

12 Jelinek T, Nothdurft HD, Rieder N, Löscher T. Cutaneous myiasis: review of 13 cases in travellers returning from tropical countries. *Int J Dermatol* 1995;34:624-6.

21 Persistent insect bites

C.L.M. van Hees

21.1 INTRODUCTION

Travellers to tropical or subtropical countries almost inevitably encounter biting and stinging insects. Such an encounter usually leads to an annoying itchy urticarial papule, which disappears in a few hours or days. Persistent insect bites or papular urticaria do not disappear for weeks to months or come and go for long periods after the original bite or bites. Flare-ups may be precipitated by new bites elsewhere on the skin. A generalised response shows numerous pruritic papules, often occurring in crops, always with excoriations and these are easily secondarily infected. The actual terminology for these conditions remains somewhat unclear although it now appears to be generally accepted that papular urticaria are a hypersensitivity response to arthropods. In this chapter I will use the term persistent insect bite for the persisting or recurring lesion at the site of a bite, the term papular urticaria for the response consisting of numerous pruritic papules.

21.2 EPIDEMIOLOGY

Insects are found all over the world. The insects, which have most commonly been implicated in persistent insect bite reactions are mosquitoes and fleas. Others are flies, bedbugs, lice and mites, though virtually any arthropod should be considered to be able to induce persistent reactions or papular urticaria (1,2). Mosquitoes are significant for their prime role in transmission of numerous diseases such as malaria, filariasis, encephalitis, dengue and yellow fever. Approximately 3000 species of mosquito have been described. Mosquitoes have six legs, two wings, two antennae and a proboscis for sucking blood (3). Female mosquitoes are the bloodsucking insects; they need blood to be able to produce eggs. Males and females both feed on nectar. Mosquitoes breed in wet swampy areas. Any amount of still water may become a breeding ground for mosquitoes. In rural areas large rice fields but also small ponds or wells may host mosquito eggs. In urban areas any ditch, pot or gutter holding water will do. Mosquitoes will bite on exposed skin areas.

Fleas are wingless insects, which feed on birds and mammals. They cannot fly but are fast movers and may jump up from the floor to about knee-high. Fleabites therefore typically appear around the ankles and lower legs. Pets such as dogs and cats carry fleas into homes world-wide. Human fleas are also widespread, but prevail in areas of poverty.

Bedbugs hide in bed headboards, furniture, and mattresses and behind wallpaper during the day and come out at night to feed on the sleeping victim in the bed. They can travel along with their victims in clothing and other luggage.

21.3 PATHOGENESIS

The exact pathogenesis of persistent insect bite reactions and papular urticaria is still unclear. Several immune mechanisms have been implicated. Both immediate and delayed hypersensitivity reactions play a role. Skin tests with deer ked extract in 5 patients with persistent reactions to deer ked bites showed positive delayed reactions in all patients, and immediate reactions in three patients. All six controls were negative (4). Penneys (5) studied circulating IgG antibodies to mosquito salivary gland proteins in relation to intensity of exposure to mosquitoes in 13 individuals. In those with a history of little or average exposure antibody binding was found; in those with extensive exposure little antibody binding was found. This seems to correlate with the skin reactions where massive exposure to mosquito bites at an early age leads to tolerance. Heng et al (6) found immunoglobulin and complement deposits in the skin of three patients with papular urticaria suggesting a role for immune complexes in the pathogenesis, with complement activation initiated through the classical pathway. Jordaan and Schneider (7) did not find immunoglobulin or complement deposits in their group of 30 patients.

There are however, distinct stages in mosquito- and fleabite immunity which have been consistently described by several authors (5,8):

1 A 5 to 7 day induction phase without symptoms.
2 Initiation of delayed hypersensitivity. After a few weeks pruritic papules or vesicles appear within a day after a fresh bite and may persist for weeks.
3 Immediate hypersensitivity (IgE-mediated) consisting of urticarial wheals within 30 minutes after a bite, followed by a late delayed reaction consisting of pruritic papules which may persist for weeks. The delayed reaction gradually fades leaving.
4 An immediate reaction only, and
5 ultimately a lack of reaction (tolerance).

Children between the ages of 2 and 7 world-wide go through these phases as they meet insects, respond to them and develop tolerance (9). After developing tolerance they will respond to repeated bites in the same way as most adults. They only develop a transient wheal but do not develop persistent papules. When persistent insect bites or papular urticaria develop in travellers they have presumably been exposed to insect antigens which were new to them and start their response in stage 1, in contrast to the more commonly occurring immediate response to familiar insects. Unfortunately in travellers it is often impossible to identify the offending insect.

Travellers returning home from a 2 or 3 week holiday will often state that their itchy rash started on the way home or during the last few days of their holiday. This correlates with development stages described above. In many of them the next few weeks are symptomatic and the reaction then fades leaving them free of symptoms presumably because contact with the offending insect has ceased. The reaction may recur upon returning to the same area. In some people the lesions persist or keep flaring up for months to years after returning home however. Calnan (10) postulates that this may be due to occult continued exposure, cross-sensitivity to another antigen, or continued presence of the allergen (saliva, broken off mouthpart) in the skin.

21.4 CLINICAL PICTURE

The immediate response to an insect bite consists of the classic wheal and flare reaction. A typical persistent insect bite presents as a pruritic urticarial papule located on exposed skin (figure 21.1).

The papule may be 2 to 10 mm in diameter. Sometimes a (micro)-vesicle surmounts the papule. Bullous reactions also occur. Larger lesions may appear as plaques. In papular urticaria numerous erythematous urticarial papules are found in clusters or groups, often on exposed skin (figure 21.2), or in a generalised distribution (figure 21.3).

Figure 21.1 *Persistent insect bite recurring on the arm of a traveller two weeks after returning from Thailand*

Figure 21.2 *Multiple itchy pruritic papules on arms and legs of a 57-year-old woman upon return from a holiday in Zambia and Malawi*

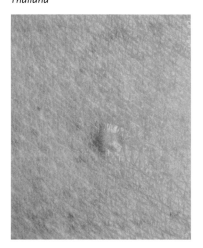

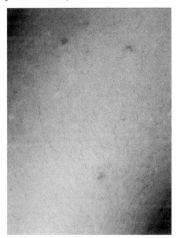

Because of severe itchiness the lesions are often excoriated. In time the papules become firm and hyperpigmented (figure 21.4).

Longstanding severely itching persistent insect bites may progress to prurigo nodularis. Scratching in warm and humid climates easily leads to bacterial superinfection with *Staphylococcus aureus* or *Streptococcus pyogenes* (figure 21.5).

When travellers have excoriated insect bites on the lower legs, a long flight home, with resulting edema of the lower legs, may delay healing (11). Large ulcers may be the result (figure 21.6).

In immunocompromised patients such as AIDS patients and patients with chronic lymphocytic leukaemia very severe papulo-vesicular and bullous, delayed and persistent, reactions to insect bites have been seen (12,13).

Figure 21.3   Papular urticaria in a Tanzanian toddler

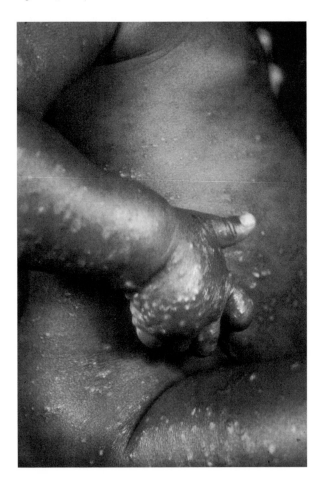

Histopathology

Jordaan and Schneider (7) studied the histopathologic features of lesions in 30 child-ren with papular urticaria in South Africa. More than 50% of their cases showed mild acanthosis, mild spongiosis, exocytosis of lymphocytes, mild subepidermal edema, extravasation of erythrocytes, a superficial and deep moderately dense mixed inflam-matory cell infiltrate and interstitial eosinophils. They stress that the histopatholo-gic features of papular urticaria are not specific, and describe four histopathologic variants; lymphocytic, eosinophilic, neutrophilic and mixed variants. Garcia et al (8) studied the histopathologic features of papules and wheals in 45 Colombian patients and found a mainly perivascular and superficial inflammatory infiltrate with mixed population of mononuclear cells and granulocytes, mainly eosinophils. The wheals and papules could not be differentiated histologically. Rantanen (4) studied 11 skin biopsies from 19 patients with persistent pruritic papules from deer ked bites. The lesions were between one day and 4½ months old. All showed an insect bite reaction; a marked dermal mononuclear infiltrate with various admixtures of eosinophils, so-metimes reaching the subcutis. Plasma cells and macrophages were frequent, espe-cially in old papules. The histological features are consistent with persistent insect bite reaction.

21.5 TREATMENT AND PREVENTION

In treatment of persistent insect bites and papular urticaria one should aim to
1   Provide symptomatic relief.
2   Identify and remove the offending insect.
3   Prevent recurrence.

Treatment can be extremely difficult. Symptomatic relief is gained primarili with topical corticosteroïds. Single bites are mostly treated with potent corticosteroïds, or milder ones under occlusion. When this is not effective intralesional corticostero-ids, excision or cryotherapie may be tried. Papular urticaria may, to some extent, re-spond to antihistamines, especially sedative antihistamines. Topically lotions or gels

Figure 21.4   Longstanding persistent insect bites with lichenification and hyperpigmentation

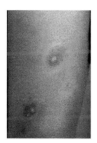

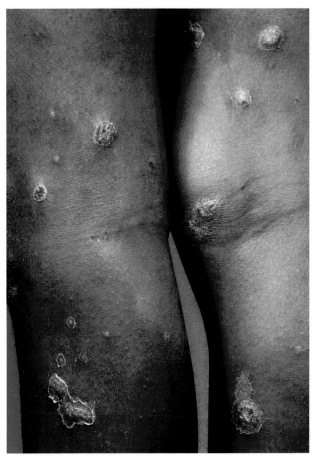

Figure 21.5   Excoriated insect bites with bacterial superinfection

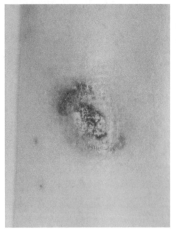

Figure 21.6   Ulcerating excoriated insect bite, infected with staphylococcus aureus, which enlarged steadily after the flight home from Senegal

containing menthol, camphor and/or pramoxine which may be compounded with topical corticosteroïds provide some relief of pruritus, as may doxepin 5% cream. For extensive lesions with severe itch a short course of systemic corticosteroïds is sometimes required. Oral antibiotics are needed in superinfection. Despite these options lesions may persist and cause severe pruritus. Beacham and Kurgansky (14) successfully treated two patients with psoralens plus ultraviolet (PUVA) therapy; Millikan (15) used a modified Goeckerman-type regime. In analogy to treatment options for nodular prurigo Naafs (16) suggests thalidomide and cyclosporin in severe recalcitrant cases.

Identifying the offending insect in travellers is very difficult. People will usually remember being bitten but often have no idea what actually bit them. The distribution pattern of the lesions on the body may be helpful. Millikan (15) proposed the following diagnostic patterns: Bites found on exposed areas may be caused by mosquitoes, flies, gnats, scabies and other mites. Bites on ventral surfaces by mites other than scabies and bugs. Bites around elastic areas of clothing by ticks, bugs and lepidoptera (moths). Household pets may carry fleas. Bedding and clothing may harbour bedbugs. These should be sought and exterminated. If local insects are responsible for the ongoing reaction prevention of bites is essential.

Protection from insect bites is best achieved by wearing protective clothing. In mosquito-infested areas avoiding being outside from dusk till dawn helps. Insect repellents containing N,N-diethyl-3-methylbenzamide (DEET) are considered by far the most effective protection against insect bites by several authors. A comparative study of insect repellents by Fradin and Day (17) found DEET extremely effective against mosquito bites on the arms of 15 volunteers, the duration of the repelling effect rising along with the concentration of DEET. A 23.8% formulation protected for an average of 5 hours, DEET 6.65% for almost 2 hours. In comparison citronella preparations did not protect for longer than 20 minutes. All tested repellent containing wristbands were useless. Pyrethrum-containing scented coils are slightly effective but dependent on environmental factors like the wind. In this study there was no comparison with picaridin (KBR 3023)-containing insect repellents, because these were not available in de Unites States. They are however widely used in Europe (in the Autan range of products) and elsewhere. Field studies in Burkina Faso (18,19) and Australia demonstrated that these products are at least as effective against mosquitoes as DEET containing formulations. DEET has been used and tested for 50 years and appears to have the broadest spectrum of effectiveness. It is effective against all insects e.g. mosquitoes, flies, mites and fleas and many arthropods including ticks. It is available in formulations ranging from 5% to 95%. When used according to the manufacturers instruction, DEET in its current formulation is considered safe to use, even in children, in doses ranging from 10 to 30% depending on the length of time exposure is expected. Instructions include once daily application,

application to exposed skin only (no occlusion), no direct application to hands and face, and washing the product off when returning indoor. The lowest feasible concentration should be used because of reported serious neurotoxic side effects (20).

REFERENCES

1 Demain JG. Papular Urticaria and Things that Bite in the Night. *Curr Allergy Asthma Rep* 2003;3:291-303.

2 Steen CJ, Carbonaro PA, Schwartz RA. Arthropods in dermatology. *J Am Acad Dermatol* 2004;50(6): 819-42, quiz 842-4. Review.

3 Goddard J. Physician's guide to arthropods of medical importance. Boca Raton CRC Press 2003. ISBN 0-8493-1387-2.

4 Rantanen T, Reunala T, Vuojolahti P, Hackman W. Persistent pruritic papules from deer ked bites. *Acta Derm Venereol* 1982;62:307-11.

5 Penneys NS, Nayar JK, Bernstein H. Circulating antibody detection in human serum to mosquito salivary gland protein by avian biotin peroxidase. *J Am Acad Dermatol* 1988;18:87-92.

6 Heng MC, Kloss SG, Haberfelde GC. Pathogenesis of papular urticaria. *J Am Acad Dermatol* 1984;10:1030-4.

7 Jordaan H, Schneider JW. Papular urticaria: A histopathologic Study of 30 Patients. *Am J Dermatopathol* 1997;19:119-126.

8 Garcia E, Halpert E, Rodriguez A. Immune and histopathologic examination of fleabite induced papular urticaria. *Ann Allergy Asthma Immunol* 2004;92:446-52.

9 Stibich AS, Schwartz RA. Papular urticaria. *Cutis* 2001;69:89-91.

10 Calnan CD. Persistent insect bites. *Trans St Johns Hosp Dermatol Soc* 1969;55:198-201.

11 Zeegelaar J, Feijter A. de, Vries H de, Lai A Fat RTM, Neumann HAM, Faber WR. Microcirculatory changes in travellers to a tropical country. *Int J Dermatol* 2002;41:93-5.

12 Davis MD, Perniciaro C, Dahl PR, Randle HW, Mc Evoy MT, Leiferman KM. Exaggerated arthropod-bite lesions in patients with chronic lymphocytic leukemia: a clinical, histopathologic and immunopathologic study of eight patients. *J Am Acad Dermatol* 1998;39:27-35.

13 Penney NS, Nayar JK, Bernstein H, Knight KW. Chronic pruritic eruption in patients with acquired immunodeficiency syndrome associated with increased antibody titers to mosquito salivary gland antigens. *J Am Acad Dermatol* 1989;21:421-5.

14 Beacham BE, Kurgansky DK. Persistent bite reactions responsive to photochemotherapy. *Br J Dermatol* 1990;123:693-4.

15 Millikan LE. Papular urticaria. *Semin Dermatol* 1993;12:53-6.

16 Naafs B. Tropical holiday memories. *Eur J Dermatol* 1999;9:500-6.

17 Fradin MS, Day JF. Comparative efficacy of insect repellents against mosquito bites. *N Engl J Med* 2002;347:13.

18 Constantini C, Badolo A, Ilboudo-Sanogo E. Field evaluation of the efficacy and persistence of insect repellents DEET, IR3535, and KBR 3023 against *Anopheles gambiae* complex and other Afrotropical vector mosquitoes. *Trans R Soc Trop Med Hyg* 2004;98:644-52.

19 Frances SP, Van Dung N, Beebe NW, Debboun M. Field evaluation of repellent formulations against daytime and nighttime biting mosquitoes in a tropical rain-forest in Northern Australia. *J Med Entomol* 2002;3:541-4.

20 Roberts JR, Reigart JR. Does anything beat DEET? *Pediatr Ann* 2004;33:443-53.

22 *Beetle dermatitis*

P. Schmid-Grendelmeier and S. Haug

P. Schmid-Grendelmeier and S. Haug

22.1 INTRODUCTION

Cutaneous reactions to contact with beetles are common problems in many parts of the world. Although not life-threatening, such reactions can be very annoying, in some cases there are also very painful lesions with secondary scarring. Blistering beetle dermatitis is the most common distinctive, seasonal vesiculobullous skin disorder that occurs some hours after contact with beetles (figure 22.1) (1).

Beetles (Order: Coleoptera) are the largest group of insects with at least 350 000 species. Only a few are relevant in human medicine.

Figure 22.1 Beetle dermatitis knee with crushed culprit (Cameroon)

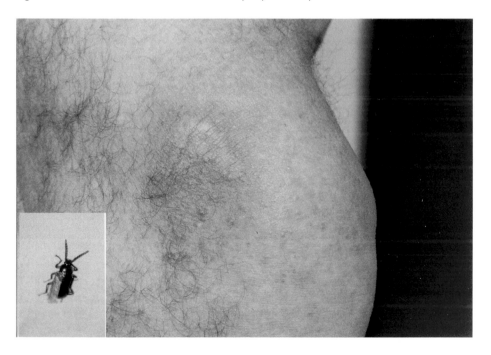

Table 22.1   Overview of human pathogenic beetles and their relevance in human medicine

	Polyphaga			Adephaga	
Family	Meloidae	Oedemeridae	Staphulimidae (rove beetle)	Hydradephaga	Geadephaga
Genus(Example)	• Lytta vesicatoria (Spanish fly) • Mylabris • Epicauta	• Heliocis repanda • Oxycopis thoracica • Ditylus • Diasclera	• Paederus fuscipes litoralis • Oxytelus tetracaninatus	• Dytiscidae • Amphizoidae • Hygrobiidae • Haliplidae	• Carabidae • Trachypachidae
Features	Adults are rather soft-bodied, long-legged beetles with the head deflexed, fully exposed, and abruptly constricted behind to form an unusually narrow neck, the pronotum much narrower at the anterior end than the posterior and not carinate (keeled) laterally, the forecoxal cavities open behind.	Prothorax is widest in the front half, narrowing towards the elytra. The elytra are parallel sided and often finely ridged. The antennae are threadlike but are slightly saw-toothed in a few species.	While they have wings and are able to fly, they have a tendency to crawl and run, resulting in a superficial similarity to ants. P. cruenticollis and P. australis have with other Paederus species bright bands of orange color over the prothorax and middle of the abdomen.	Adults with notopleural sutures visible on prothorax, with six visible abdominal sterna, the first three fused and divided by hind coxae; pygidial defense glands.The body forms of some have become highly modified structurally for life in unusual habitats (e.g., gyrinids at the air-water interface, paussine carabids in ants' nests, rhysodines in heartwood).	
Venom	Cantharidin		Paederin	Adephagans are fantastic producers of chemicals in a variety of forms. Thesechemical characters are, for the most part, clearly understudied in many groups.	
Toxic effect	Cantharidin penetrates the epidermis readily and produces violent superficial irritation, resulting in vesication a few hours later. If sufficient quantities are absorbed topically, renal dysfunction may result (14).		Highly toxic alkaloid, which causes acute dermatitis after 12-36 with burning senstions, erythema and blistering.		

Beetle dermatitis is mainly caused by three major groups of beetles (see also table 22.1):

- Meloidae.
- Oedemeridae.
- Staphylinidae.

The prothorax of beetles is generally very distinct while the two posterior thoracic segments are more or less fused to the abdomen. The life cycle of beetles involves larval and pupal stages before emergence of the adult. Many beetles feed on plants throughout their life cycle, many are predators or scavengers and a few are parasitic. Several families have toxic secretions that may be deposited on the skin.

The majority are of medium size (15 mm) and have soft leathery forewings (elytra).

22.2 EPIDEMIOLOGY AND GEOGRAPHIC DISTRIBUTION OF BEETLES INDUCING SKIN REACTIONS

22.2.1 Meloidae
The archetype for blister beetle dermatitis is the eruption produced by species of the family Meloidae. More than 200 species are known to produce blister beetle dermatitis and these are distributed worldwide (2). The most notorious of the meloid blister beetles is *Lytta vesicatoria* (Linnaeus), the 'Spanish flySpanish fly', which is found in Southern Europe in the summer when blister beetle dermatitis occurs.

The majority is of medium size (15 mm) and has soft leathery forewings (elytra).

22.2.2 Oedemeridae
The least known family to cause BBD is the Oedemeridae. In contrast to reports of Meloidae the reports of oedemerid BBD are limited to the Pacific Basin and the Caribbean. Approximately 1500 species of Oedemeridae are found worldwide (3) and are attracted by white light.

22.2.3 Staphylinidae
Staphylinidae (rove beetles) is the largest of these families, containing at least 26 000 species worldwide. Within this family, members with vesicating properties are limited to the genus *Paederus*, numbering several hundred species. These insects are widely distributed over the continents of Europe, Africa, South America, Asia and Australia. Rove beetles are slender elongated insects ranging from 5 mm to 10 mm length. While they have wings and are able to fly, they have a tendency to crawl and run, resulting in a superficial similarity to ants. When disturbed, they commonly arch their abdomen up over their body in a scorpion-like posture. These beetles feed

on decaying vegetables and animal matter and are also predatory on other small insects. They are also attracted to white lights at night, a feature that commonly brings them into contact with humans.

In Australia, *Paederus* species are widespread in rural areas and two members have been proven to cause vesicular eruptions, *P. cruenticollis* and *P. australis*.

A large outbreak was recognized in central coastal Queensland, Australia,with a conservative estimate of 250 cases in late 1998. Other series of beetle dermatitis are reported from the Arizona desert (USA during heavy rain and flooding) (4), Iran with an annual outbreak of *Paederus* dermatitis (PD) in the summer months (5) and Turkey between May and July 1997 (6).

22.2.4 Adephagan beetles

The coleopteran suborder Adephaga contains eight families, all of which secrete a variety of glandular substances. All families possess paired pygidial glands located postero-dorsally in the abdomen. The suborder Adephaga represents a taxonomically well-defined group of beetles which exhibit a wide variety of chemical secretions and associated behaviors and ecological interactions. Although a great deal of information on adephagan chemistry is available, no publications thoroughly address the entire suborder.

Apart from the interesting nature of the chemistry of these beetles, an understanding of the components of their glands could provide insight into relationships and evolutionary history of families within the group. The taxonomy and systematics of adephagan families is not yet well resolved.

All Adephaga deliver compounds in one of three ways depending on taxon. These are

1 oozing,
2 forceful spraying,
3 crepitation.

The glands of many groups are not equipped with muscles for discharging large amounts of substance (such as the prothoracic glands in *Dytiscidae*). For this reason, these groups are only capable of more limited expulsion of compounds and the material oozes out from the openings. This is in part facilitated by turgor pressure and by indirect action of nearby muscles. In contrast, many groups, most notably *Carabidae*, have intrinsic muscles directly associated with the glands. In this case, secretions can be ejected with varying amounts of force depending on taxon.

Pasimachus subsulcatus was found to be capable of forcibly discharging a spray of several centimeters (7). The final type of delivery, crepitation, is limited to the brachinine lineage of *Carabidae* and its near relatives. This well-known phenomenon has led them to be called bombardier beetles. They can be found in middle Europe.

Not all insects within each of these families are capable of producing blisters.

The adults of most species appear to be obligate pollen feeders and are thus commonly found on flowers.

22.3 PATHOMECHANISMS AND CLINICAL APPEARANCE OF BEETLE DERMATITIS

Blister beetle dermatitis is clearly an important cause of blistering eruptions due to mostly toxic effects. So a toxic-irritative dermatitis is the most commonly seen clinical feature. The dermatitis is due to a potent and highly irritant vesicant contained in the body fluids of such beetles, which is released if the beetle is brushed, pressed, or crushed against the skin (8). Usually beetles do not have a bite or sting venomous to humans. The patient may be unaware of contact with the insect because the primary contact with the beetle is painless and seldom remembered by the patient. An overview of cutaneous reactions is given in table 22.2. The reactions are listed in the various modes of skin contact and pathophysiologic responses.

22.3.1 Meloidae, Oedemeridae, Staphylinidae

By far the most common manifestation of beetle-induced reactions in human beings is blister beetle dermatitis, so subsequent we will concentrate on this.

Initial contact is painless and so goes unnoticed. The lesions are erythemato-vesicular to start with, but within a day or two turn necrotic, giving rise to a burnt or charred appearance. Symptoms like burning, itching and pain are almost always associated. A characteristic feature is the development of kissing lesions, where a blister comes into contact with another area.

Table 22.2   Clinical features of cutaneous reactions

	Toxic (Cantharidin, Pederin)	Toxic by hair of pillars	Allergic	Stings or bites	Transferred disease
Example	· Meloidae · Oedemeridae · Staphylinidae	· Dermestes	· Zabrotes subfaciatus · Trogoderma angustum (Dermestidae)	· Coccinella septempunctata · Coccinella undecimpunctata · Dytiscus marginales	· Tribolium castaneu · Tenebrio molitor · Dermestes peruvianus · Stegobuim paniceum · Melolontha
Clinic	blister beetle dermatitis	histamine liberaration on the affected skin area	allergic rhinitis and conjunctivitis	injuries caused by bites	intermediate host of Hymenolepis diminuta and Hymenolepis nana

22.3.2 Meloidae, Oedemeridae

As both the Meloidae and Oedemeridae (3) contain cantharidin, the eruptions produced are similar. The blistering agent cantharidin is an odorless terpene (exo-1.2-*cis*-dimethyl-3.6-ep-oxyhexahydro-phthalic anhydride). Contact with these substances causes no reaction or pain initially. Inflammation due to cantharidin usually occurs within 2-3 hours. Cantharidin then causes itchy blisters on exposed skin which are often linear. Localized erythema over 2 to 3 hours resulting from contact with the swatted or crushed bug and the release of toxin and irritation are the first findings (9). Then a red rash occurs which blisters in 2-4 days associated with increasing pain (10). There is a large variation in individual susceptibility to blistering from cantharidin; some subjects never blister despite heavy exposure. It heals in one week but may remain itchy for some time. Post inflammatory hyperpigmentation can persist for months.

If cantharidin is taken internally it produces profound gastrointestinal irritation (2). The mechanism of action of cantharidin involves the release or activation of neutral serine proteases that act specifically on the dense desmosomal plaque (11). The progressive disappearance of the dense desmosomal plaque leads to the detachment of tonofilaments from desmosomes with the appearance of acanthoysis and an intra-epidermal blister. The action of cantharidin is entirely epidermal and lesions heal without scarring.

Recorded cantharidin content of adult beetles (by dry weight) ranges from less than 1% to a high of 5.4%.

The lesions of oedemerid BBD appear to be smaller than those of meloid BBD because most oedermerid species are smaller then meloids.

22.3.3 Staphylinidae

The clinicopathologic picture of *Paederus* (Staphylinidae) BBD differs because these beetles produce a different chemical, paederinpaederin a highly toxic alkaloid.

Crushing *Paederus* beetles on the skin has no immediate effect as well, but in clinical experience and observations acute dermatitis appears 12-36 hours later, corresponding in shape and dimension to the area over which the substance was released.

Clinically the sudden onset of stinging and burning sensations accompanied by micropustules on erythematous bases characterizes PD. Linear lesions, kissing ulcers and drip marks are among the useful diagnostic clues. The duration of PD in typical cases is 1-2 weeks but in some cases the duration was much longer and it may remain itchy for some time. Post inflammatory hyperpigmentation can persist for months.

Ocular involvement is relatively common finding usually secondary to transfer of the toxic chmecal from elsewhere on the skin by the finger (5) and presents usually with unilateral perorbital dermatitis, but some cases have severe periorbital edema and sometimes you even find a keratoconjunctivitis, which has been named 'Nairobi eye' (12). Pederin results in cutaneous eruptions of a greater severity than those produced by cantharidin. This substance differs from cantharidin in its biologic, physical, and chemical properties. *Paederus* BBD is characterized by a more violent cutaneous reaction with prominent urtication and dermatitis prior to blistering (1).

Due to its delayed appearance, the rash is not often linked to the insect, so only a small number of patients identified the cause.

Patients often remembered having been outdoors during the previous day but only a minority had noticed the beetles or suspected them as being causal. Several patients recalled walking through a spider web before developing the rash. Patients usually had no knowledge of the whiplash rove beetle, but some presented already aware of the diagnosis, most commonly referred to as 'acid beetle' dermatitis. Patients likened the sensation to a burn.

All age groups can be affected. Lesions predominantly affect exposed areas especially the face, neck, shoulders and forearms. Sporadic lesions are also reported on the chest and abdomen. Most lesions are linear and affect only one area of the body. Blisters are usually described as being multiple and minute although found many cases with bullae up to 1 cm of diameter.

Systemic upset, mucosal or conjunctival involvement is found in only a few anecdotic cases (12).

Healing occurs in approximately 10 days. Pruritus is common during this time. The majority of lesions resolve without complication but secondary infection and post-inflammatory hyperpigmentation were common.

22.4 DIAGNOSTIC PROCEDURES

Diagnosis is mostly made by the clinical history and the typical cutaneous lesions. However, histopathology may provide useful information. The diagnosis may even be suggested, particularly in the early stages of the lesion when extensive epidermal necrosis with prominent exocytosis of neutrophils and incipient intraepidermal vesiculation with an intact stratum. In many areas there was almost full-thickness epidermal necrosis with a variably intact basal layer and suprabasal blister formation. In some areas even the basal layer can be destroyed. Rarely, epithelial necrosis extends down the superficial aspect of hair follicles to the level of the sebaceous duct. There is also a moderate perivascular and interstitial infiltrate of lymphocytes and histiocytes in the superficial and mid-dermis. Neutrophils are also present superficially and associated with papillary edema. Only a rare eosinophil is seen. Oedemerid BBD produces histopathologic findings identical to meloid BBD.

Exposure to pederin causes a spectrum of histopathologic changes, ranging from epidermal necrosis and blistering in the acute stages to marked acanthosis with mitotic figures in the late stages. PD is an entomologic model of irritant contact dermatitis, having histophatologic features of intraepidermal and subepidermal blistering, epidermal necrosis and acantholysis (5).

The histologic features of arthropod bites are usually less extensive and more focally arranged, and include superficial and deep perivascular and periadnexal lymphocytic infiltrates with eosinophils scattered among collagen bundles. The presence of some acantholytic foci relatively far from the foci of clinically involved skin suggests a possible indirect role of pederin in inducing acantholysis, probably through the release of epidermal proteases (13).

A lesion of intermediate duration reveals epidermal hyperplasia with mild basal spongiosis and regenerative changes associated with necrosis of superficial keratinocytes, neutrophil exudate and focal parakeratosis. A moderate superficial lymphohistiocytic infiltrate can be present and papillary edema remains.

A late lesion reveals a superficial layer of necrotic epidermis with overlying intact stratum corneum. This is separated from the underlying regenerated epidermis by a narrow cleft representing the resolved blister. Only a sparse superficial perivascular mononuclear inflammatory cell infiltrate is present.

The number of people affected during an outbreak such as the one in Australia assists in establishing the diagnosis; however, sporadic isolated cases may occur during the year for which a correct diagnosis may not be made. In these cases, only a single lesion may be present and it may not have a classical linear or mirror image appearance.

22.5 PREVENTION AND TREATMENT

Insecticides are an efficient – however not always very environmentally-friendly way – to reduce the number of insects including beetles. In densely populated buildings such as hospitals it can be sometimes absolutely mandatory to treat rooms with such insecticides as otherwise real epidemics of beetle dermatitis can occur. Repellents, which by definition are used to move arthropods away from the host, are effective in avoiding beetle contact only to a certain extent. An effective way to prevent beetle contact, at least during the night, is the use of mosquito nets treated with insecticides as used very effectively in the prophylaxis of malaria also.

There is no specific treatment available due to the toxic nature of the lesions. Treatment of lesions was attempted with potent topical corticosteroids, antibiotics, acyclovir and antihistamines. All these treatments were minimally effective and are purely symptomatic. Antibiotics are needed for secondary infection and topical corticosteroids and systemic antihistamines are helpful in cases with severe itch. In many cases also analgesics are needed due to the sometimes very strong pain related to the skin lesions.

REFERENCES

1   Alexander JOD. Arthropods and human skin. Berlin: Springer Verlag, 1984:81-2.
2   Lehmann CF, Pipkin JL, Ressmann AC. Blister beetle dermatosis. *Arch Dermatol* 1955;71:36-8.
3   Arnett (II). The false blister beetles of Florida (*Coleoptera: Oedemeridae*). Entomology Circular: Florida Department of Agriculture and Consumer Service Division of Plant Industry 1984;259:1-3.
4   Claborn DM, Polo JM, Olson PE, Earhart KC, Sherman SS. Staphylinid (rove) beetle dermatitis outbreak in the American southwest. *Mil Med* 1999;164(3):209-13.
5   Zargari O, Kimyai-Asadi A, Fathalikhani F, Panahi M. *Paederus* dermatitis in northern Iran: a report of 156 cases. *Int J Dermatol* 2003;42:608-12.
6   Sendur N, Savk E, Karaman G. *Paederus* Dermatitis: A Report of 46 cases in Aydin, Turkey. *Dermatology* 1999;199:353-5.
7   Davidson BS, Eisner T, Witz B, Meinwald J. Defensive secretion of the carabid beetle Pasimachus subsulcatus. *J Chem Ecol* 1989;15:1689-97.
8   Nicholls DS, Christmas TI, Greig DE. Oedermerid blister beetle dermatosis: A review. *J Am Acad Dermatol* 1990;22:815.
9   Kerdel-Vegas F, Goihman-Yahr M. *Paederus* dermatitis. *Arch Dermatol* 1966;94:175-85.
10   Southcott RV. Injuries from *Coleoptera*. *Med J Aust* 1989;151:654-9.
11   Bertaux B, Prost C, Heslan M, Coulomb B, Dubertret L. Cantharide acantholysis: endogenous protease activation leading to desmosomal plaque dissolution. *Br J Dermatol* 1988;118:157-65.
12   Poole TR. Blister beetle periorbital dermatitis and keratoconjunctivitis in Tanzania. *Eye* 1998;12:883-5.
13   Borroni G, Brazzeli V, Rosso R., Pavan M. Paederus fuscipes dermatitis: a histopathological study. *Am J Dermatopathol* 1991;13:467-74.

23 Aquatic skin disorders

M.T.W. Gaastra

M.T.W. Gaastra

23.1 INTRODUCTION

More than 70% of our earth is covered with water. For that reason it is not strange that more dermatoses related to the aquatic environment are seen by dermatologists and other doctors. Due to the increase in modern mobility with low fare rates, people tend to travel to more exotic places for leisure aquatic activities or to practice aquatic sports. Also there is a demographic trend to move to coastal areas. Another fact is that people wear less protection when it comes to bathing suits. Marine creatures have the most potent venom known to humans; some are life threatening. For this reason it is important to recognize the cutaneous and systemic symptoms in order to make a correct diagnosis and give adequate treatment. Aquatic dermatology is not taught in residency training programs. The first major book was published in 1978 by Fisher and Oris: 'Atlas of Aquatic Dermatology'. In 1985 Mandojana and Letot published Dermatologie Aquatique. In 1987 an issue of *Clinics in Dermatology* was dedicated to aquatic dermatology. The chapters were written by 29 contributors. Williamson published in 1987 'The Marine stinger guide' which gave excellent information about the aquatic creatures in the Australian area. Mandojana was the first to attempt to get a systemic approach in the field of aquatic dermatology. They are ordered to the type of mechanism (e.g. sting, bite) involved (1).

I   Irritation (Contact dermatitis).
   A   Direct chemical (allergic and toxic); jellyfish, chlorinated water, sponges, algae, sea cucumbers, sea moss, fish, etc.
   B   Diving gear: irritant, allergic, and toxic.
II   Infection.
   A   Primary: cercarial dermatitis or 'swimmer's itch' (*Schistosome* species).
   B   Secondary: bacteria (*Pseudomonas* species), mycobacterioses (*Mycobacterium marinum*), bacilli (*Erysipelothrix* species), *Vibrio* species, algae (*Prototheca* species) and other miscellaneous infections.
III Wounds.

    A   Active: stings (hydroids, Portuguese man-of-war ,shells (cones), punct-ure, and suction (cephalopods (Octopi) wounds, (annelids (leeches) and abrasion (elasmobranches: manta ray skin), etc.

    B   Passive: abrasions and cuts (corals), punctures (fish spines, spiny crea tures (echinodermis)), spiculous creatures (sponges), bristly creatures (worms), etc.

IV   Hypersensitivity reactions: aquagenic urticaria, aquagenic pruritus of the elderly, aquagenic pruritus, and 'bath itch' (polycythemia rubra vera).

V   Aquatic sports-related lesions: 'swimmer's ear', water-ski cord strangulation of extremities, etc.

VI   Dermatitis by ingestion: scrombroid fish (tuna, etc.) and ciguatera (usually by large tropical fishes).

VII   Bites.

    A   Serious: destructive (sharks, moray eels, etc.) and venomous (sea snakes, etc.)

    B   Other: fishes, worms, sea lice, and miscellaneous.

VIII Barotrauma: mask and diving suit squeeze.

IX   Electric shock: fresh water electric eels, etc.

In the following pages the most important and most frequently occurring aquatic dermatoses will be shortly discussed.

23.2 CNIDARIAN ENVENOMATIONS

The phylum Cnidaria (formerly known as coelenterata) encompasses 3 major classes:

1   Scyphozoa (jellyfish).

2   Hydroxoa: (hydroids, 'fire-coral', Portuguese man of war').

3   Anthozoa: (sea anemones and hard and soft corals).

Cnidarian stings are the most frequently encountered injuries in the aquatic envi-ronment. Thus far 9000 cnidarian species have been identified. All of them share the same envenoming organ. The nematocyst consists of a sack-like structure (cnido-blast) filled with venom and a coiled thread (figure 23.1).

The nematocyst can be activated by direct pressure or by changes in the direct environment. The thread penetrates the entire epidermis and the venom is directly delivered in the papillary dermis. Because of this the venom is quickly brought into the circulation. Nudibranchs and octopi that eat cnidariae use the intact nematocysts for their own protection and bring them to their skin. Tentacles broken after a storm and that float free can still sting humans. The sea bather's eruption is caused by these free floating parts (2). The venom consists mainly of toxic or antigenic proteins and

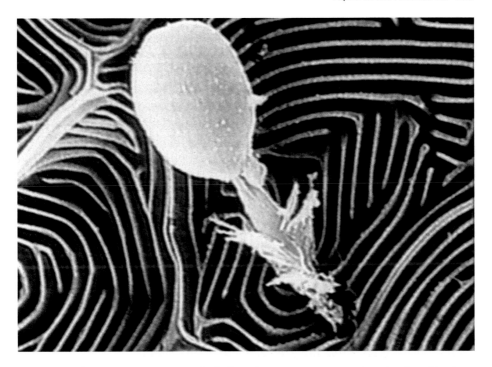

Figure 23.1   Electronmicroscopic image of a discharged nematocystnematocyst entering the epidermis

enzymes (collagenase, proteases, elastases, nucleases, hyal-uronidase and phospha-tase). Other are histamine, histamine-releasers, serotonin and kinine-like substances (3,4). The most common immediate symptom of a jellyfish sting is an acute local dermatitis: a linear, urticarial erythematous eruption that follows the pattern of the contact of the tentacles. The lesions can be necrotizing or ulcerative. A burning pain or a pruritic sensation can be felt. Depending on the species the forming of long lasting and scarring skin lesions can occur (figure 23.2).

Recurrent eruptions from jellyfishjellyfish stings are frequently reported lasting from several months up to a year. The most venomous jellyfish is the *Chironex fleckeri* (south-east pacific jellyfish). It is found in the northern and western parts of Australia (figure 23.3).

Full thickness necrosis can occur in several days after contact. Other systemic reactions can lead to haemolysis, acute renal failure, cardiac and respiratory arrest. Fatalities may occur in 10-20% of the *C. fleckeri* stings. An antivenom is available for *C. fleckeri* envenomations (5). From a dermatological point it is important to treat the eruption with potent steroids (sometimes even systemic) to prevent chronic reactions and postinflammatory hypo- or hyperpigmentation with severe scarring or atrophy. Secondary infection by aquatic bacteriae is not uncommon.

Systemic reactions

Some jellyfish can provoke systemic, toxic reactions. This may include headache, malaise, weakness, diaphoresis and lacrimation. Less common are ataxia, dizziness, fainting, local cramping, muscle spasms, convulsions, paresthesias, arthralgia, chills, vomiting, diarrhea, blurred vision, throat constriction, respiratory depression and coma. The best way is to avoid the contact with these organisms. Wearing special protective clothing can make a big difference in the contact (5,6). During the

Figure 23.2   Months after Chironex fleckeri contact

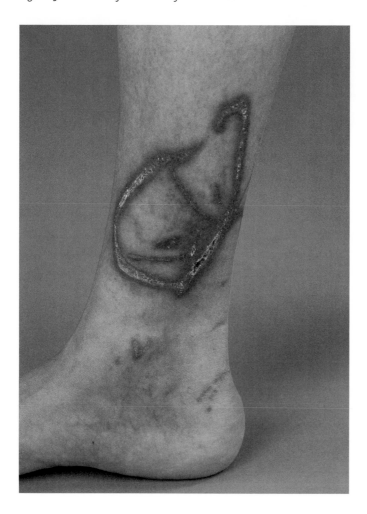

Chironex season in Australia beaches are protected by special nets. The public is well informed when there are sightings (figure 23.3).

Treatment

Avoid further nematocyst discharge and immobilize the extremity. The inactivation of the nematocysts is best done by pouring vinegar (4-6% acetic acid) on the afflicted area for at least 30 seconds. Some authors promote the use of meat tenderizer although its effectiveness has never been established. Most of the venoms are thermolabile. For that reason apply local hot water (42-45 °C). Remove the tentacles with a raiser or C-card. Check the ABC's (airway, breathing and circulation) and treat the systemic reactions with epinephrine, corticosteroids and antihistamines (2,5,6).

Figure 23.3   Warning sign in Jellyfish stinger season

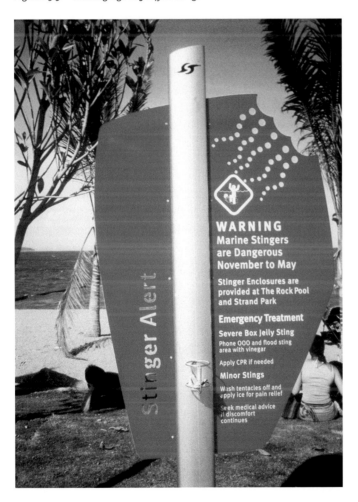

Hydrozoa and Anthozoa can cause a milder stinging sensation with erythematic and swelling. In a later stage papular urticaria, hemorrhage, morbilliform rash and vesicular and pustular formation. In the case of 'fire coral' (*Millepora* spp.) not only the burning sensation can occur but also cuts from the hard lime carbonate skeleton can cause serious wounds (7,8).

23.3 SPONGE DERMATITIS

A variety of species can produce irritation when in contact with the skin. They cause this by their sharp silica spicules or by irritation like 'glass wool'. A number of sponges are toxic. Two syndromes can occur after sponge contact.

1   Pruritic dermatitis (like plant allergic contact dermatitis). The most well known sponge that causes this is the 'fire sponge' *(Tedania ignis)* which is found in the Hawaiian and Caribbean islands. In general within a few hours the skin becomes pruritic and burns. Afterwards it appears mottled and purpuric. Most reactions subside within 3-7 days. Sometimes fever, chills, malaise, dizziness, nausea and muscle cramps occur.

2   Irritant contact dermatitis from the penetrations of the silica spicules. Severe cases can develop into an exfoliative dermatitis. There is no really effective treatment. Potent steroids provide the most benefit but they have no effect on the initial toxic reaction. Soak the affected area in vinegar (4-6% acetic acid) and use topical disinfectants (8)

23.4 SEAWEED DERMATITIS

Lyngbya majuscula is a subtropical seaweed well known for its acute toxic reaction. After storms dislodged fragments of seaweed enter bathing suits. The victim develops a stinging, burning or pruritic sensation within minutes or hours. In the swimming suit area escharotic blistering may develop. After washing with water and soap low potency steroids are helpful. The eruption usually subsides within a week (6,8).

23.5 PRIMARY INFECTIONS

Cercarial dermatitis

This is a maculopapular cutaneous eruption caused by a *Schistosoma* species, in cercarial form derived from blood flukes that infect animals. Only a short exposure is necessary to penetrate the skin. An intense pruritic papular dermatitis of 7-10 days ensues (1,6,8).

Sea bather's eruption

It has many causative agents. Most are cnidarian nematocysts. It can occur in covered or in exposed skin. After 4-24 hours after exposure a mild macular dermatitis to a maculopapular or vesicular eruption can form. Sometimes systemic reactions occur that are similar to the ones found after cnidarian contact (figure 23.4). Delayed reactions are reported. Symptomatic treatment remains the best option for both conditions (1,6,8).

23.6 SECONDARY INFECTIONS

Erysipelothrix rhusiopathiae is a gram positive, facultative aerobic bacillus that can survive for months. The infection it causes is known as 'fish handlers disease', 'seal finger', 'speck finger' or 'erysipeloid of Rosenbach'. It is known as an occupational hazard. A mild dermatitis occurs 1-7 days after a wound. There is an edematous halo circumscribed by a centrifugally advancing, raised, well demarcated, and marginated

Figure 23.4   Sea bather's eruption

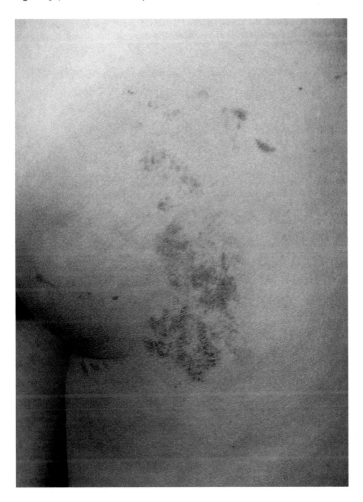

erythematous ring around the central area. If untreated the reaction will usually run its course in 1-3 weeks. Sometimes arthritis, septicemia or endocarditis may occur. Aqueous penicillin G is given i.v.

Vibrio vulnificus is a particularly virulent marine *Vibrio* (gram negative, free living bacterium). It is found in water temperatures between 13-20 °C. They are natural habitants. The infected area rapidly becomes erythematous, edematous and painful, with fast spread of the cellulitis to the adjacent areas. Hemorrhagic vesicles or bullae develop at the site of primary infection. A period of necrotizing vasculitis follows that turns into necrotic ulcers (figure 23.5).

 Other signs include fever-like chills and sepsis. *Vibrio vulnificus* is highly fatal by septic shock. *Vibrio parahaemolyticus* can produce similar life-threatening syndromes with necrotizing myonecrosis. After a rapid diagnosis the initial treatment with the adequate antibiotic is essential. The antibiotics of first choice are trimethoprim-sulfamethoxazole or ciprofloxacin.

Aeromonas hydrophila (gram negative) is found in fresh water. A puncture wound may become cellulitic in 8-24 hours with erythema, edema and purulent discharge.

Figure 23.5 Infected wound after hard coral contact (Vibrio alginolyticus)

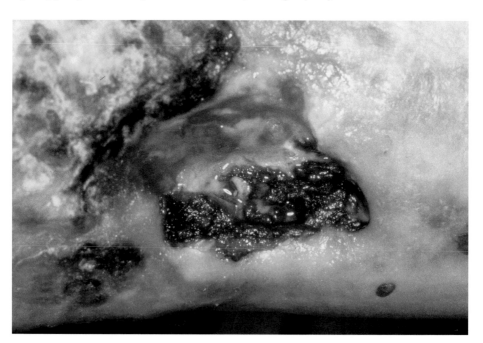

It may resemble typical streptococcal cellulitis. The same antibiotics can be used as described by the vibrio infections.

Chromobacterium violaceum is a gram negative rod that is found in (sub)tropical fresh water rivers. The skin symptoms are secondary to bacteriaemia leading to diffuse pustular dermatitis, vesicles, ecchymatic maculae, macupapular rash, subcutaneous nodules, ulcers and cellulitis. It is sensitive to trimethoprim – sulfamethoxazole (1,6,8).

23.7 VENOMOUS AND NON-VENOMOUS FISH STINGS AND WOUNDS

23.7.1 Sting rays
Wounds are either lacerations or punctures. Pain is immediate. Systemic reactions may occur. Thorough irrigation is useful, but never close the wound by sutures. Antibiotic prophylaxis may be used.

23.7.2 Barracudas (Sphyraena spp.) and moray eels
Barracudas (Sphyraena spp.) and moray eels are not aggressive. Both may strike if they are disturbed. They can hold or strike and release. The wounds must be well irrigated with fresh water. Antibiotic prophylaxis can be useful (7).

Figure 23.6   Sea urchin granulomas

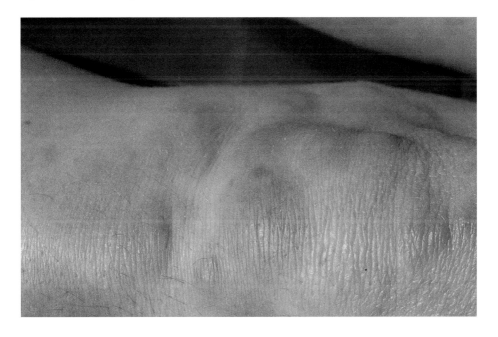

23.7.3 Echinoderm (sea urchins, star fish) injuries

Echinoderms are benthic invertebrates with a radical, symmetric collomate body. There are 3 classes (Echinoidea, Halothurioidea, Asteroidea). There are hundreds of species of the sea urchin. In some species the spines, that are mostly located on the upper surface, are tipped with poisonous glands. Envenomation can also be caused by the seizing organs (pedicellariae) on the lower surface. People step on sea urchins or brush against them. This causes several puncture wounds which can be extremely painful. The broken spines remain embedded or leave the skin unbroken. A 'tattooing' pattern is frequently seen. Most of the fragments are absorbed after a while or eliminated through the epidermis. If the spines enter near a joint, destruction and synovitis can occur. In the skin the development of foreign body granulomas is a regular finding after these injuries (1,6,7) (figure 23.6).

If there is any doubt as to the diagnosis, an x-ray of the joint is useful. The spines are radio opaque. The therapy is symptomatic. Several therapies are advised by local people but their use has never been proven in studies. The *Acanthaster planci* (crown of thorns) is the most venomous tropical starfish (*Asteroidea*). They produce an acute painful puncture wound or a chronic swollen lesion with lymphadenopathy. Their spines are as hard as wood. Frequently these injuries are complicated by infection. Wounds need to be doused with vinegar or isopropylalcohol and afterwards placed in non-scalding hot water (42-45 °C) (6,7).

Bristle worms (Phylum: Annelida; Class: Polychaeta) have rows of thin, chitinous bristles that grow from the lateral parts of their bodies. When a worm is disturbed the bristles become erect. They penetrate the skin like polyester spines. Some of these are venomous. A pruritic, erythematous, papular and edematous eruption can develop with a burning sensation. Necrosis and paresthesias are rare. The wounds are self-limited but secondary infection is not rare. Remove the bigger bristles with a forceps and the smaller ones with adhesive tape. After this, use vinegar (4-6% acetic acid). For persistent inflammatory reactions topical steroids may be useful (1,7).

As stated in the introduction the field of the aquatic dermatology is a growing one and it is not possible to highlight all the aquatic dermatoses. For that reason a brief overview of the most frequently encountered aquatic dermatoses has been presented.

REFERENCES

1 Mandojana RM. Introduction to Aquatic Dermatology. In: Joseph Demis D, (ed.). Clinical Dermatology 23rd edition. Philadelphia: Lippincott-Raven, 1996: 8-29 A+B.

2 Burnett JW, Calton GJ, Burnett HW. Jellyfish envenomations syndromes. *J Am Acad Dermatol* 1986;14:100-6.

3   Burnett JW. Human Injuries following jellyfish stings. *MMJ* 1992;41:509-13.

4   Burnett JW, Calton GJ. The chemistry and toxicology of some venomous pelagic Coelenterates. *Toxicon* 1977;15:177-96.

5   Fenner PJ, Williamson JA. Worldwide deaths and severe envenomations from jellyfish stings. *Med J Aust* 1996;165:658-61.

6   Fenner PJ, Williamson JA, Burnett JW. Clinical aspects of envenomations by marine animals. *Toxicon* 1996;34:145.

7   Auerbach PS. Envenomation by aquatic Invertebrates. In: Auerbach PS. Wilderness medicine, 4th edition. St. Louis: Mosby, 2001:1450-87.

8   Auerbach PS, Halstead BW. Injuries from non venomous aquatic animals. In: Auerbach PS. Wilderness Medicine, 4th edition. St. Louis: Mosby, 2001:1418-49.

General references

Angelini G, Bonamonte D. Aquatic Dermatology. Milano: Springer – Verlag Italia, 2002.

Fisher AA. Atlas of Aquatic Dermatology. New York, Grune & Stratton, 1978.

Mandojana RM (guest ed). Aquatic Dermatology. Clin Dermatol 1987:5(3).

Williamson JA, Fenner PJ, Burnett JW, Rifkin JF. Venomous and poisonous marine animals. Sydney: University of New South Wales press, 1996.

24 Geographic distribution

This chapter correlates the geographical distribution with the skin diseases acquired during travel. These tables can be consulted, and can be helpful in establishing a diagnosis.

Table 24.1 Climatic zones with associated skin diseases

Rainy	Monsoon	Semi-arid	Arid
bacterial infection	bacterial infection	photodermatoses	photodermatosies
superficial fungal infection	superficial fungal infection	veld sore	desert sore
persistent insect bite	persistent insect bite	cutaneous diphtheria	scorpions, spiders
subcutaneous myiasis	creeping eruption	cutaneous leishmaniasis	bristles, spikes, thorns
dengue	dengue	rickettsioses	
		scorpions, spiders	
		bristles, spikes, thorns	

Table 24.2 Common skin diseases from South and Middle America

Travellers	Immigrants
persistent insect bite	scabies
cutaneous leishmaniasis	subcutaneous mycosis
cutaneous larva migrans	mycobacterial skin disease
tungiasis	leprosy
larva currens	HIV related skin disease
aquatic dermatoses	
pyoderma	
dengue	

Table 24.3 Common skin diseases from Africa

Travellers	Immigrants
persisent insect bite	scabies
myiasis	subcutaneous mycoses
cutaneous larva migrans	mycobacterial skin disease
tungiasis	leprosy
cutaneous leishmaniasis	lymphatic filariasis
onchocerciasis	onchocerciasis
schistosomiasis	trypanosomiasis
lymphatic filariasis	HIV related skin diseases
beetle dermatitis	
spider bites	
pyoderma	
cutaneous diphtheria	
rickettsial fevers	
trypanosomiasis	

Table 24.4 Common skin diseases from Middle East and India

Travellers	Immigrants
persistent insect bites	lymphatic filariasis
scorpion stings/spider bites	mycobacterial skin diseases
cutaneous leishmaniasis	leprosy
pyoderma	HIV-related skin diseases
rickettsial fever	
aquatic dermatoses	

Table 24.5   Common skin diseases from Southeast Asia

Travellers	Immigrants
persistent insect bite	mycobacterial skin diseases
cutaneous larva migrans	leprosy
larva currens	HIV-related skin diseases
gnathostomiasis	aquatic dermatoses
schistosomiasis	
dengue	
typhoid	
pyoderma	

Table 24.6   Common skin diseases from Australia and Oceania

Travellers
persistent insect bite
aquatic dermatoses
spider bites

25 Clinical problems

When suspecting an imported skin disease the reader can consult one of the following flow charts. The charts present a symptomatic approach; with the following clinical entities:

1 itch;
2 ulceration;
3 fever and rash;
4 eschar;
5 nodular lymphangitis;
6 diagnosis of leprosy.

Figure 25.1 Itch

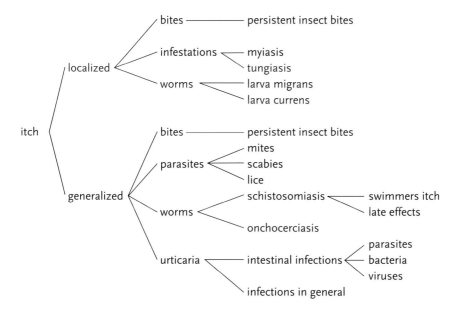

Figure 25.2   Ulceration

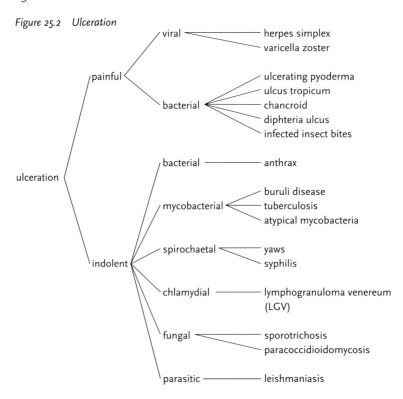

Figure 25.3   Fever and rash

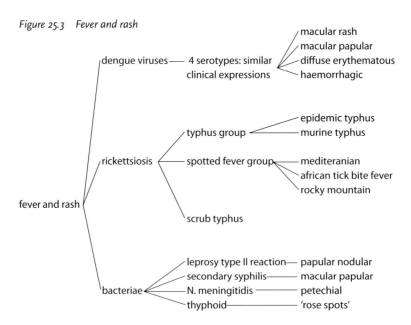

Figure 25.4   Eschar

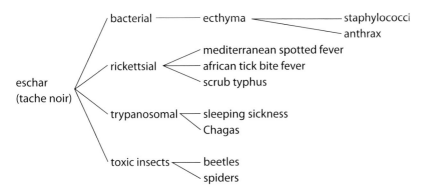

Figure 25.5   Nodular lymphangitis

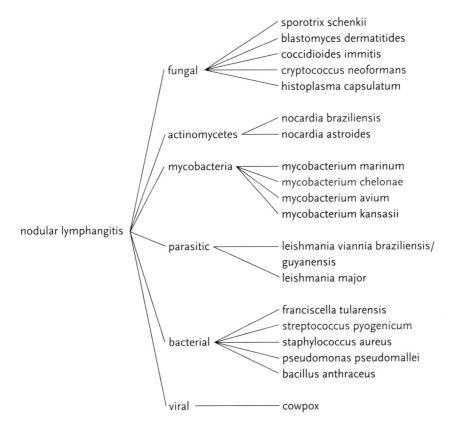

Figure 25.6   Diagnosis of leprosy

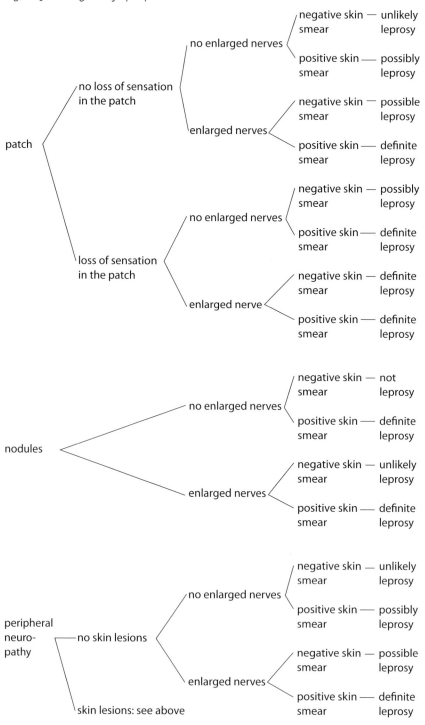

Acknowledgement illustrations

Chapter 2: The figures are from the authors.

Chapter 3: The figures are from the author, some are originally from the Departments of Dermatology, Erasmus University, Rotterdam (photographer J. van der Stek) and Academic Medical Center, Amsterdam (photographer B. Vrees), the late prof.dr. D.L. Leiker, The Netherlands and the Regional Dermatology Training Centre, Moshi, Tanzania.

Chapter 4: The figures are from the Departments of Dermatology, St Franciscus Gasthuis (photographer J. Kool) and Erasmus University, Rotterdam (photographer J. van der Stek).

Chapter 5: The figures are from the editors, some are originally from the late prof. dr. D.L. Leiker, The Netherlands, P.L.A. Niemel, Surinam, the Departments of Dermatology, Erasmus University, Rotterdam (photographer J. van der Stek) and Academic Medical Center, Amsterdam (photographer B. Vrees), the Regional Dermatology Training Centre, Moshi, Tanzania and the Instituto Lauro de Souza Lima, Bauru Brazil.

Chapter 6: The figures are from the Department of Dermatology Academic Medical Center and the Department of Dermatology, Erasmus University, Rotterdam (photographer J. van der Stek).

Chapter 7: The figures are from the author, some are originally from the Department of Dermatology Erasmus University, Rotterdam (photographer J. van der Stek) and the Academic Medical Center, Amsterdam (photographer B. Vrees), the late prof.dr. D.L. Leiker, The Netherlands and the Regional Dermatology Training Centre, Moshi, Tanzania.

Chapter 8: The figures are from the author.

Chapter 9: Figure 9.4 is from W.M. Meyers, Armed Forces Institute of Pathology, USA.

Chapter 10: Figure 10.5 is from M. Brakman, Reinier de Graaf Groep location Delft, The Netherlands.

Chapter 11: Some of the figures are from P.P.A.M. van Thiel, Academic Medical Center, Amsterdam.

Chapter 12: The figures are from the author.

Chapter 13: The figures 13.3-13.6 are from Perine P.L., Hopkins D.R., Niemel P.L.A., St. John R.K., Causse G., Antal G.M. Handbook of Endemic Treponematoses. Yaws, Endemic Syphilis and Pinta. World Health Organization, Geneva, 1984, used with permission of the World Health Organization. The figures 13.1, 13.2 are from the collection of J. van der Stek, Rotterdam.

Chapter 14: The figures are from the authors and the Department of Dermatology, Academic Medical Center, Amsterdam, The Netherlands.

Chapter 15: The figures are from the author and the Departments of Dermatology, Academic Medical Center, Amsterdam and Leiden University Medical Center, Leiden, The Netherlands.

Chapter 16: Figure 16.1 is from World Health Organization, http://www.who.int/pbd/blindness/onchocerciasis/ocp/en/; http://www.who.int/pbd/blindness/onchocerciasis/apoc/en/; http://www.who.int/pbd/blindness/onchocerciasis/america_map/en.
Figure 16.2 is from Laboratory-confirmed reports to the Health Protection Agency, Communicable Disease Surveillance Centre (CDSC), Colindale, London – as of 23rd November 2004.
Figure 16.4 from Murdoch M.E. The skin and the immune response in onchocerciasis. *Tropical Doctor* 1992;22 (suppl 1):44-55.

Chapter 17: The figures are from the Department of Dermatology, Erasmus University, Rotterdam (photographer J. van der Stek), The Netherlands.

Chapter 18, 19 en 20: The figures are from the authors.

Chapter 21: The figures are from the author; figure 21.4 from the late A.H. Verhagen, The Netherlands; figure 21.5 from Department of Dermatology Leiden University Medical Center (fotographer H. Korff), The Netherlands.

Chapter 22: The figures are from H.C. Koppert.

Chapter 23: The figures are from the author.

Index